THE
EVERYTHING®
GUIDE TO
NOOTROPICS

Dear Reader,

It is my pleasure to write *The Everything® Guide to Nootropics*. As a
nutritional therapist, personal trainer, and nutraceutical educator, I have
worked with many clients who needed different things to improve
their brain health and mental performance. When I noticed a continually decreasing ability to focus on schoolwork while I was in college, it
became the wake-up call that inspired me to become an expert in what's
considered "alternative therapies" for improving cognitive function.

After recovering my own cognitive function, I've been on the journey
to help millions pull themselves out of a mental slumber and take charge
of their lives again. If you don't have the ability to think clearly and efficiently, you are sabotaging your potential success in life. As the world
speeds up and competitiveness reaches new heights, you'll need all the
mental firepower you can get.

Nootropics will always be a big part of my life. As I wrote this book,
I learned much more than I anticipated. The world of optimal brain
health will always remain somewhat elusive. The brain is a wonderful
thing!

Evan Brand, NTP, CPT

Welcome to the EVERYTHING® Series!

These handy, accessible books give you all you need to tackle a difficult project, gain a new hobby, comprehend a fascinating topic, prepare for an exam, or even brush up on something you learned back in school but have since forgotten.

You can choose to read an Everything® book from cover to cover or just pick out the information you want from our four useful boxes: e-questions, e-facts, e-alerts, and e-ssentials.

We give you everything you need to know on the subject, but throw in a lot of fun stuff along the way, too.

We now have more than 400 Everything® books in print, spanning such wide-ranging categories as weddings, pregnancy, cooking, music instruction, foreign language, crafts, pets, New Age, and so much more. When you're done reading them all, you can finally say you know Everything®!

QUESTION

Answers to common questions

FACT

Important snippets of information

ALERT

Urgent warnings

ESSENTIAL

Quick handy tips

PUBLISHER Karen Cooper

MANAGING EDITOR, EVERYTHING® SERIES Lisa Laing

COPY CHIEF Casey Ebert

ACQUISITIONS EDITOR Hillary Thompson

DEVELOPMENT EDITOR Eileen Mullan

EVERYTHING® SERIES COVER DESIGNER Erin Alexander

Visit the entire Everything® series at *www.everything.com*

THE
EVERYTHING®
GUIDE TO
NOOTROPICS

Boost your brain function with smart drugs
and memory supplements

Evan Brand, NTP, CPT

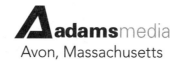

Avon, Massachusetts

*To my family and friends who have always encouraged
me to chase my dreams and break the status quo.
I've written this book because of you.*

Published by
Adams Media, a division of F+W Media, Inc.
57 Littlefield Street, Avon, MA 02322. U.S.A.
www.adamsmedia.com

Contains material adapted from *The Everything®
Wild Game Cookbook* by Karen Eagle, copyright
© 2006 by F+W Media, Inc., ISBN 10: 1-59337-545-
X, ISBN 13: 978-1-59337-545-4; *The Everything®
Lactose-Free Cookbook* by Jan McCracken,
copyright © 2008 by F+W Media, Inc., ISBN 10:
1-59869-509-6, ISBN 13: 978-1-59869-509-0; *The
Everything® Cast-Iron Cookbook* by Cinnamon
Cooper, copyright © 2010 by F+W Media, Inc.,
ISBN 10: 1-4405-0225-0, ISBN 13: 978-1-4405-0225-
5; *The Everything® Green Smoothies Book* by Britt
Brandon with Lorena Novak Bull, copyright ©
2011 by F+W Media, Inc., ISBN 10: 1-4405-2564-
1, ISBN 13: 978-1-4405-2564-3; *The Everything®
Paleolithic Diet Book* by Jodie Cohen and Gilaad
Cohen, copyright © 2011 by F+W Media, Inc.,
ISBN 10: 1-4405-1206-X, ISBN 13: 978-1-4405-1206-
3; *The Everything® Eating Clean Cookbook* by
Britt Brandon, copyright © 2012 by F+W Media,
Inc., ISBN 10: 1-4405-2999-X, ISBN 13: 978-1-4405-
2999-3; *The Everything® Giant Book of Juicing* by
Teresa Kennedy, copyright © 2013 by F+W Media,
Inc., ISBN 10: 1-4405-5785-3, ISBN 13: 978-1-4405-
5785-9; and *The Everything® Wheat-Free Diet
Cookbook* by Lauren Kelly, copyright © 2013 by
F+W Media, Inc., ISBN 10: 1-4405-5680-6, ISBN 13:
978-1-4405-5680-7.

ISBN 10: 1-4405-9131-8
ISBN 13: 978-1-4405-9131-0
eISBN 10: 1-4405-9132-6
eISBN 13: 978-1-4405-9132-7

Printed in the United States of America.

10 9 8 7 6 5 4 3 2 1

This book is intended as general information
only, and should not be used to diagnose
or treat any health condition. In light of the
complex, individual, and specific nature of
health problems, this book is not intended to
replace professional medical advice. The ideas,
procedures, and suggestions in this book are
intended to supplement, not replace, the advice
of a trained medical professional. Consult your
physician before adopting any of the suggestions
in this book, as well as about any condition that
may require diagnosis or medical attention. The
author and publisher disclaim any liability arising
directly or indirectly from the use of this book.

Always follow safety and commonsense cooking
protocol while using kitchen utensils, operating
ovens and stoves, and handling uncooked food.
If children are assisting in the preparation of
any recipe, they should always be supervised by
an adult.

*This book is available at quantity discounts for
bulk purchases. For information, please call
1-800-289-0963.*

Contents

Acknowledgments

Thanks to my wife for giving me the courage, confidence, and most importantly, the delicious food every evening to keep my brain fueled enough to write this book. I couldn't have done it without you . . . literally!

Introduction

NOOTROPICS ARE DRUGS, SUPPLEMENTS, nutraceuticals, and foods that can enhance your cognition and boost your brainpower. Are you feeling dazed and confused, like you are in a mental fog? Are you having trouble concentrating on important tasks? Nootropics can help.

The world of nootropics is where marketers, scientists, and health enthusiasts all converge. The term "nootropics" hasn't been around for long, and the true meaning of "nootropic" has already been diluted. There are now hundreds of supplement companies popping up across the globe with the intention of not only making a profit, but also claiming to help people to perform at a level higher than the average non-supplemented human. This book will show you how to use these brain enhancers to refocus your attention on your personal, career, and financial goals.

You are about to embark on an incredible look into the world of ancient medicine and modern science. There have been relatively little changes to the physical framework and requirements of human DNA for eons. Human beings have always (and will always) require nourishment of the mind, body, and spirit to be healthy, happy, and functional. Luckily, technology has made this goal more accessible. In fact, most of the compounds you will discover in this book can be purchased either at your local supplement store or on the Internet and shipped right to your door.

Without a solid foundation of diet, lifestyle, and exercise, your human potential is limited. You will soon discover that the perfect recipe for a positive life is optimal cognitive performance, a healthy weight and metabolism, and the right supplements. These days, with prescription drugs, energy drinks, and caffeine abuse, people are burning the candles at both ends and they are doing it quickly.

You don't have to wear yourself out. Nootropics can naturally revitalize your nervous system and make you a calm and collected human, just as you were designed to be. Let the fast-paced world speed past you, as you become more efficient in less time. The goal of this book is to show you how to work smarter, not harder. You are only given a specific amount of time in life. It is the most valuable possession you have, next to your mind and body. Use that time wisely.

CHAPTER 1

Using Nootropics to Boost Your Mind

In this technological age, people care more about productivity and speed than ever before. They are overscheduled and overworked, and are looking for a way to do more in the same number of hours in the day. What if there were ways to create more efficiency in the hours that you are working? What if you were told that success in your personal and business life isn't about how hard you work, but how smart you work? Nootropics can become your secret weapon to change the way you think and perform when it comes to your everyday life and tasks.

What Are Nootropics and Smart Drugs?

Nootropics comes from the Greek words *nous* and *trepin*, which roughly translates as "to bend the mind." While bending the mind sounds slightly frightening, understanding that your mind is supposed to be flexible is a key component to understanding how to improve your creativity, efficiency, and overall cognitive ability.

Nootropics and smart drugs can be sourced from natural or synthetic sources for the intention of enhancing your creativity, energy, attention, and cognitive ability; for preventing neurodegeneration and protecting brain cells; for enhancing sleep and mood; for increasing physical performance; for allowing new patterns of thought; and much more.

Researchers are increasingly talking about a term called "neuroplasticity," which simply means that you can change your brain over time. Habits, addictions, and other things that may seem set in stone are actually quite malleable. People who have been burdened with mental illness or just a slight cognitive deficit may be able to reverse their conditions and improve their brain function over time.

Nootropics can't make you operate like you've seen in the movies, where a character takes a pill and can remember an entire encyclopedia in one sitting, but they can play a key role in helping you gradually enhance your ability to focus, think clearly, and be more productive.

While the rest of the world attempts to fuel themselves with caffeine and sugar for a quick-lived rocket-fuel type of boost, people who invest their time and energy into discovering a nootropic nutrient that works for them can improve their abilities, functions, and quality of life.

ALERT

The definitions of "nootropic" and "smart drugs" have become vague and confusing in recent years. Nootropics are supposed to refer to substances with no side effects or toxicity. Some smart drugs may be prescribed only by a physician and can have various side effects and other potential downsides. Companies may use either of these terms in their marketing efforts, so you should use your best judgment.

History of Nootropics and Smart Drugs

Since the definitions of "nootropics" and "smart drugs" have similarities, these two terms may be used interchangeably throughout this book. Typically, smart drugs are referring to synthetic creations that come from a laboratory and give a cognitive effect. Nootropics can refer to synthetic materials as well, but as you'll discover later in this book, there are many "earth-grown nootropics" that could be grown right in your backyard to give you the effects you desire.

Mankind has constantly sought improvement of brain function and has sought out mind expansion and psychedelic states for eons. From cave paintings in France that date back thousands of years to the stories of monks using meditation and certain plants to enhance their practice, it's obvious that humans have craved a sense of enhancement for many years.

Green Tea as a Nootropic

One of the longest-used nootropics is the plant *Camellia sinensis* var. *sinensis*, more commonly known as green tea. Historical records and folklore discuss the use of green tea as an aid to achieve deeper states of consciousness, especially during meditation practices. Due to an amino acid called L-Theanine that will be discussed later, the act of drinking certain teas can enhance a certain brain wave to aid in increased concentration and attention while reducing fatigue and stress.

The more popular and potent version of green tea is called matcha. This is a special type of green tea that is shaded from the sun for about three weeks before harvest. When you shade the plant, the levels of theanine are increased. Matcha is a ground powder made from these shaded green tea leaves. It is mixed directly into the hot water and consumed in its entirety. This allows you to absorb and assimilate more nutrients than you would normally receive from a tea made by infusion.

During the Tang Dynasty in China (618–907), pulverized tea was documented. Later, during the Song Dynasty (960–1279), mixing tea that was a ground powder with hot water in a bowl became popular. Little did these tea consumers know that they were drinking a tea that would take nearly a thousand years to become trendy.

Cognitive Enhancement Across Cultures

Matcha isn't the only ancient ingredient that has been used for cognitive enhancement and productivity. In the Amazon region of Ecuador, the Huaorani people, also known as the Waos, use various plants and poisons derived from frogs to enhance their cognitive ability and eyesight to aid them during hunts. You may recall seeing the application of frog poison to a tribesman's eyes on a BBC documentary called *Human Planet*, a series that documents the miraculous feats that humans achieve across the planet. While frog poison doesn't fit into the typical classification requirements of a nootropic today, it is an interesting example of a way humans have enhanced their performance in their survival tasks.

Many Native American cultures still use different plant medicines for celebratory and ritualistic acts today. You'll learn what the "true requirements" of a nootropic are a little bit later, but for now, understand that humans have been pushing the boundaries of performance and consciousness this way for longer than you can imagine. This is partially what allowed such rapid and unfathomable advancements in civilization and the species as a whole.

ESSENTIAL

Nootropics and cognitive enhancers in general can come in many shapes, sizes, and application methods such as powders, capsules, tablets, and liquids. You may drink, swallow, or even sniff a compound to get the desired effect, as in the example of essential oils and other aromatic materials. Matcha tea is the perfect example of an aromatic and liquid nootropic-consumption experience.

Tapping Into Ayurveda

The field of Ayurveda, a system of natural healing that is alive and strong today, has been around for nearly 5,000 years and combines the use of herbs, minerals, plants, and other ingredients to heal ailments, enhance cognitive function, and more. This is an increasingly popular topic around the yoga community since the intersection between mindfulness, physical activity, and natural medicine has emerged.

The Benefits of Ginkgo Biloba

The *Ginkgo biloba* tree is considered a living fossil since it has much in common with samples dating from the Permian period 270 million years ago. This tree is native to China and has been cultivated by monks since about 1100 A.D. for its many medicinal benefits.

For many years the ginkgo was thought to be extinct, but in 1691 German naturalist Engelbert Kaempfer discovered the tree alive and well in Japan. Its popularity and cultivation migrated to the Western world, and ginkgo is now used in many dietary supplement formulas to enhance brain function and support general cognitive ability.

This book will help you understand and cultivate a deeper appreciation for the natural world that offers so many unique plants, herbs, and nutrients that can help mankind. It makes you wonder if they were "put there" for human beings to use, or if it's merely a coincidental occurrence. Whatever you believe, the undeniable and scientifically validated compounds you are about to learn about have the potential to change your life forever. Whether your intention is to make a million dollars with your new business idea, or if you just want to have more energy and focus to take care of your family, you will soon have a nootropic toolbox guaranteed to rock your world.

Nootropics 101

"Nootropic"—the modern term for brain-enhancing compounds—was coined by the Romanian psychologist and chemist, Dr. Corneliu E. Giurgea. He coined the term in 1972, just eight years after he synthesized piracetam, the world's first synthetic nootropic.

To earn the term nootropic, he stated that compounds should have the following characteristics:

1. They should enhance learning and memory.
2. They should enhance resistance against learned behaviors such as electric shock and hypoxia (lack of oxygen).
3. They should protect the brain against various physical or chemical injuries, such as those incurred by pharmaceutical drugs.
4. They should possess very few side effects and have extremely low toxicity.

5. They should increase the efficacy of the tonic cortical/subcortical control mechanisms, leading to an improvement in both conscious and subconscious behaviors.

Natural versus Synthetic

There are both natural and synthetic compounds that can be considered nootropics. The term "nootropic" is used very loosely; many different compounds are marketed as nootropics although they don't fit the desired parameters set by Dr. Giurgea. The information in this book may be seen as a dilution of the term, but for lack of a better word it will refer to different nutrients in various compounds as nootropics.

Some may possess cognitive enhancing effects, while others may reduce stress and increase your ability to calm down. With recent marketing trends, the word "natural" denotes safer and more efficient products than the word "synthetic." When it comes to smart drugs and discussing brain-enhancing nutrients, however, the science is what determines the safety.

If you are on the hunt for natural herbs and plants, the word "natural" is a good start. However, with industrial pollution from China reaching epidemic levels, you must verify that the quality of the soil that the plants were grown in was healthful and not full of heavy metals and other toxic chemicals.

ALERT

Just because something is natural doesn't make it healthy. There are plenty of 100 percent natural mushrooms in the wild that can cause severe illness and even death. Similarly, synthetic compounds do not automatically lose all credit for those living a "natural" lifestyle. There are many synthetic compounds that are completely safe and effective at boosting your brain function, without the need for fear.

Many seasoned health seekers purposely avoid sourcing any ingredient, especially nootropics, from China because of pollution. However, Chinese people have been cultivating some of these nutrients for millennia and have a particularly beneficial and potent method for obtaining the highest quality available. In these cases, it just makes sense to source from China. Other compounds can be grown successfully and healthfully in North America, where third party testing for heavy metals, other contaminants, and verification of ingredient potency is readily available.

Dealing with Modern-Day Stressors

Soil depletion is a major issue plaguing even the most advanced countries, which has resulted in widespread mineral deficiencies in the population. When you are deficient in minerals, your nervous system does not have the proper conductive materials necessary to provide electrical impulses for both muscular and mental processes. You can think of minerals as the spark plugs of life. Even though you may have fuel in the form of food, sunlight, and water, if you do not have adequate mineral stores, the fuel will have trouble being converted into usable energy to power your life's activities.

FACT

Another common issue in first-world countries is depression. In fact, the Centers for Disease Control and Prevention (CDC) estimates that by the year 2020, depression will be the number one leading cause of disability in the United States. It is difficult to have a thriving economy and healthy population if mood disorders characterized by cognitive dysfunction, such as depression, continue to spread like a virus.

Impacts of Our Modern Lifestyle

Since the inception of agriculture, estimated to be around 10,000 years ago, human beings have been on a steady and general decline of overall health. While your ancient ancestors faced far higher infant mortality rates and death from infection and common injuries that could be solved today, they had a generally healthier overall experience due to the abundance of what are now called organic and natural food sources. After adopting agricultural practices that allowed civilization to flourish and grow in size, your ancestors took some necessary shortcuts to provide some sort of sustainability. In essence, it would be hard to have a modern civilization that lives a dualistic life of hunter-gatherers. Therefore, your ancestors had to make a compromise between these two vastly different ways of life to ensure optimal performance of their cognitive abilities.

In modern times, the job market is more competitive than ever. The average work week now exceeds forty hours per week, and with cell phones and e-mail available at the press of a button (or a touch screen, more accurately), there is never a time for humans to turn their brains off. This results in over-stimulation of the nervous system.

The Autonomic Nervous System

The autonomic nervous system is divided into two branches, known as the sympathetic and parasympathetic nervous system. Some time in your ancestry, your relatives would have existed in a predominantly parasympathetic state, characterized by rest, relaxation, recovery, and healing. The sympathetic mode of the nervous system, also known as the fight-or-flight system, would rarely have been engaged to help them adapt to an emergency threat such as a predator, an intruder, or a natural disaster. Humans are genetically wired to respond to these acute stressors and excel at handling them.

This sympathetic fight-or-flight response starts with the production and release of cortisol, a stress hormone that essentially cranks up all of the body's systems. Cortisol combines with other hormones (such as adrenaline) in the bloodstream to pump blood to the extremities to allow faster running, stronger arms, and a general heightened sense of awareness.

Normally, emergency situations that require this type of response only last for a few minutes or so. After that, the nervous system should switch back over to the parasympathetic state, allowing rest, recovery, digestion, and all of the other background processes that are supposed to happen. Things like wound healing, muscle building, and other restorative processes require a proper balance of parasympathetic and sympathetic nervous system activity.

For thousands of years, humans have had all of the necessary nutrients and tools needed to respond to the stressors of life, whether they were physical, mental, or emotional. However, with technological innovation has come less free time and more stress. For every push in one direction, there is a balancing act that is taking place behind the scenes. That balancing act is the field of nutrient therapy, cognitive enhancement, and the study of how natural compounds can help you adapt to this new way of life.

Dealing with Chronic Stress

Humans are not wired for chronic acute stress. (That term almost sounds like an oxymoron. It is.) Chronic stress is highly detrimental to the brain's memory center, the hippocampus. The hippocampus needs to be in a healthy and intact state for the conversion of short-term memory to long-term memory.

Cortisol is not always evil, but in the context of brain health and optimizing your cognitive performance, your cortisol levels must be under control. Cortisol is supposed to be highest in the morning to give you the energy to pursue your daily tasks, and lowest in the evening so that you can rest and recover.

The reason that modern life causes cognitive and physical deficits is because the primitive wiring system that humans are built with thinks that every input is a stressor. From the sound of a cell phone notification, to a gang of sirens parading down the street, to your boss adding unrealistic expectations and deadlines to your plate, the body never has a chance to switch over to the rest and relaxation mode.

Your parasympathetic mode must be engaged to properly assimilate the nutrients necessary to produce brain chemicals that allow you to focus. In fact, digestion is a parasympathetic process. This is partly why eating on the go and eating during or after a confrontation or other stressful event leaves you feeling hungry and unsatisfied. Your body did not have a chance to put these nutrients (assuming you are eating them) into action.

Ultimately, a healthy foundation of nutrition, movement, quality sleep, and a positive attitude can help you build a lifestyle necessary to cultivate focus, memory, attention, and, in general, the ability to handle the stresses of modern life.

Who Benefits from Nootropics?

If you mention the term "nootropic" or "smart drug" to an elderly person, he might laugh or raise his eyebrows in confusion or fear. However, in scientific research, the elderly are commonly sourced for research studies to attempt to help their cognitive decline.

At the other end of the spectrum, you have entrepreneurs and busy executives who simply want to squeeze more productivity out of the day. Both of these groups make up the steadily increasing number of people seeking alternatives to conventional medical treatment for more benign health issues such as cognitive decline, brain fog, and depression and other mood disorders.

Teachers and scientists are people who work very long hours, skip meals, and may generally live unsustainable lifestyles due to their busy schedules and passion for helping educate the population. These types of people can actually forget they need to eat because they're so focused on the task at hand, and can have a high success rate using nootropic compounds. Of course, like everything in life, these compounds are best in moderation.

These compounds are a healthy alternative to stimulants and other types of drugs. More than a decade ago, over 10,000 randomly selected college students were asked about their nonmedical use of prescription stimulants and other substances. The data collected revealed that stimulant use was present in nearly 7 percent of the student population. Prescription and non-prescription drugs for cognitive enhancement, study sessions, and for general recreational use has increased on college campuses since then.

If you know what you are doing, have a general understanding of what you're putting in your body, and have proper medical advice and guidance, you can safely enhance the function of your attention memory and overall enjoyment of life by using nootropics. Using any substance that can make you feel and perform better can be a double-edged sword, as it can become difficult to imagine life without it. The good thing about nootropic compounds is that many of them have zero risk for dependence, withdrawal, or negative side effects.

One smaller (but equally important) group of people that benefits from these compounds is brain injury victims. This group is made up of people who have suffered a variety of brain injuries, such as being subjected to loud explosions and other dangerous experiences from serving in the military, playing high school or college football, or taking repetitive hits to the head. There is an increasing amount of science that shows certain nutrients can help the brain recover from traumatic injury and other types of cognitive deficits caused from lifestyle or physical, mental, and emotional damage.

You don't have to fit into any of these categories to use nutrients and compounds to enhance your brain function. You could be a regular person who simply wants to keep focus on your kids, have more energy, improve multitasking ability, enhance your metabolism, and so on. Just because you aren't a high-powered athlete doesn't mean you can't benefit from the compounds in this book.

Are Nootropics Safe?

The next and naturally occurring question is usually "Are these things safe?" The answer is a resounding yes. Certain studies focus on a small subset of compounds discussed in this book, but many other compounds have had thousands of double-blind placebo studies done on their safety that support their validity and effectiveness. Depending on the person's biochemical individuality, diet, lifestyle, and other variables, results may vary.

One key part of using these compounds is understanding that there is an inverted U-shaped dose response curve. This means that just a little bit of a compound may be helpful, a little bit more may result in a "peak experience," but a little bit too much may result in diminished performance, anxiety, brain fog, and other symptoms that you may be trying to target. It is important to understand that if a little bit of something is good, more of that same thing might actually not be better. In a world of overconsumption and impulsive behavior, the importance of this statement cannot be emphasized enough.

When you combine two or more chemicals, nutrients, and other compounds, you may get an antagonistic or synergistic effect. For example, when discussing toxic chemicals found in plastics and other man-made containers, one chemical by itself may not be that dangerous. But if you add another chemical to that one, or, in some cases, a dozen chemicals together, you get an exponentially toxic effect. Humans are resilient by nature—otherwise they wouldn't have risen to the top of the food chain. However, with over 100,000 chemicals added to the environment in the last hundred years, a well-thought-out plan to combat and overcome the effects of these toxins is necessary for optimal brain performance.

When you combine synthetic chemicals that you are exposed to (via pharmaceutical drugs, for example), you increase the risk of toxicity. The beneficial compounds you will learn about can be helpful for preventing brain cell loss, but can also help reverse cognitive deficits and other mental disorders caused by a myriad of stressors.

Your Healthy Foundation

Supplements are designed to do exactly what their name implies: supplement. They are not a direct replacement for the raw materials that need to be obtained from your diet and lifestyle. Instead, they add to these raw materials.

All humans require the same elements to be healthy and happy. Some of the most crucial pieces of the puzzle include:

- A nutrient dense, organically grown, anti-inflammatory diet
- An adequate quantity and quality of exercise
- The right amount of sunlight exposure for both the eyes and skin
- A balance of isolation and social interaction
- The right quality, quantity, and timing of sleep

The Qualities of a Good Diet

When you hear the word diet, you might roll your eyes. The important thing to remember is that all humans have a diet. The term just represents the foods that you eat. One reason that the topic of diets, or what humans should eat, became so controversial and confusing is that just 100 years ago, 80 percent of the foods in the grocery store did not exist. From hydrogenated fats, oils, and processed and fortified grains, to the scary middle aisles of the grocery store that contain Frankenfoods, genetically modified organisms, and a plethora of carcinogenic pesticides, the food you have at your disposal now is not the same as what your ancestors ate.

In fact, it's likely that your great-grandparents lived on a farm, and that they consumed foods in their natural state, definitely close to the original source of the animal or plant itself. When automobiles became popular, people no longer had to live on a farm to get access to a variety of different foods. And now, in 2015, you could live in Buffalo, New York and get a pineapple in the dead of winter.

In 1894, Dr. Weston A. Price, founder of the National Dental Association, began to consider diet the primary factor causing tooth decay. He traveled the world to explore and study indigenous cultures and the correlation between diet and health. He discovered that cultures that ate a native diet that included properly prepared, nutrient dense foods had great health, healthy teeth, and an overall happy existence. The cultures that adopted foods of commerce that had never been present in their diets before, such as sugar and grains, suffered from growth development issues, dental issues, and other health problems. The negative health effects of modern foods on these indigenous people were amplified after multiple generations consumed them. Does this sound familiar to what's happening in the United States?

Organically raised animals positively influence your overall health, cognitive ability, and brain nourishment. Just think: Your ancestors likely consumed other parts of these naturally raised animals that are no longer popular in our culture, such as the organ meats and the brains of animals such as cows. Before you spit out your coffee, understand that bovine brain is a rich source of phosphatidylserine, a powerful nutrient for protecting human brain cells and enhancing overall cognitive ability. Without including animal protein in your diet, your potential for optimal brain performance, memory, and overall energy will be reduced.

ALERT

Nutrition is the most cost-effective way to maintain your health. Supplements range in price, but combining supplements and high-quality nutrition becomes far cheaper than the more expensive and depressing alternatives, which can involve surgery, a stack of pharmaceuticals, and a general degradation of quality and enjoyment of life.

Another key component of animal protein (such as grass-fed beef) is vitamin B_{12}, which cannot be obtained in adequate amounts from vegetables alone. Vitamin B_{12} plays a key role in the normal functioning of the brain and nervous system, and in the formation of blood. It plays a role in DNA synthesis and regulation, and also in amino acid metabolism (the nutrients that make your brain chemicals that will be discussed in later chapters). Even a slight deficiency of vitamin B_{12} can cause a wide variety of symptoms such as fatigue, depression, and poor memory.

You may hear this saying a lot, but remaining hopeful is key. The availability of organic, healthy animal and plant foods is increasing at supermarkets, farmers' markets, and corner stores across the country. Before you spend money on supplements to enhance your brain function, ensure that you have the following in your diet:

- Organic and pasture-raised meats, such as grass-fed beef, bison, venison, and pork, in moderation
- Organic fruits consisting primarily of berries for their high antioxidant value and low sugar content, including (but not limited to) blueberries, blackberries, raspberries, and strawberries
- Organic vegetables and safe starches consisting of dark leafy green vegetables for their high antioxidant value and detoxification compounds such as spinach, kale, broccoli, Swiss chard, and sweet potatoes, and white rice in moderation.
- Organic herbs and additional seasonings to enhance overall health and brain function, such as cilantro, rosemary, lavender, garlic, Himalayan salt, and pepper
- Organic healthy fats, such as avocado, butter, olive oil, coconut oil, and raw dairy, as desired or tolerated
- Spring water and organic teas, as desired
- Sweeteners in extreme moderation, such as raw honey and stevia

The truth is, there is nothing more powerful for the function of your mind and body than what is on your plate. There are no neutral foods. Every bite you take either helps or hurts your health. This is an empowering fact to keep in mind as you navigate the grocery store. You may have heard of the strategy of sticking to the perimeter of a grocery store—that's exactly the location of all the foods just listed. Prioritize quality over quantity and you will be well on your way to nourishing your mind and helping yourself and your family reach optimal performance.

Exercise Boosts the Mind

Did you know that exercise has been shown to be an equally beneficial treatment modality for major depression and cognitive deficits then commonly prescribed SSRIs? A study in the *Journal of the American Medical*

Association (*http://archinte.jamanetwork.com/article.aspx?articleid=485159*) looked at three groups of depressed patients. One group participated in an aerobic exercise program, another group was given an antidepressant, Zoloft, an SSRI, and a third group was given both. After 16 weeks, 60 percent of the exercise-only group no longer met the criteria for major depressive disorder, compared to 68 percent in the medication group. It's true. Exercise is one of the most potent medicines that you can add to your life. And it can be free! A gym membership is nice, but it's not required to simply go for a walk on your lunch breaks, before you start your day, or with your spouse or significant other after a nice evening meal.

If you go back in time to your hunter-gatherer ancestors once again, walking was a way of life. It was mandatory for survival. When the availability of cars increased, walking became an optional activity for leisure and weight reduction. MRI scans of the brain reveal an incredible amount of improvement in blood flow and cognitive performance after just a 15-minute walk. Walking is a brain-boosting supplemental activity that should be part of your daily regimen. It may take a few weeks to develop a consistent walking schedule, but after the positive benefits begin to show, you will be hooked.

American physician and cardiologist Paul Dudley White, an advocate of preventative medicine, said, "A vigorous five-mile walk will do more good for an unhappy but otherwise healthy adult than all the medicine and psychology in the world." Danish philosopher Soren Kierkegaard said, "Above all, do not lose your desire to walk. Every day, I walk myself into a state of well-being and walk away from every illness. I have walked myself into my best thoughts, and I know of no thought so burdensome that one cannot walk away from it."

Exercise has been shown to boost both healthy brain chemicals that improve your mood and cognitive function, but also boost pain relieving compounds such as endorphins. It's amazing to think that something so powerful is so commonly ignored. Walking can be one of the best habits to create on top of a solid dietary foundation.

Friends Can Help

Social isolation in adulthood is a psychosocial stressor that can result in cognitive impairments. It has been linked to a gain in body weight and shrinkage of the hippocampus, which may result in impaired memory. From an evolutionary perspective, family and friends would have been both abundant and present in the past. Now it's common to only interact with these people on a monthly, or even yearly, basis. Although "alone time" can be helpful for decompressing and relaxing at the end of a long day, skipping out on social events with others can impair your brainpower.

There are websites such as *www.Meetup.com* that allow you search for groups of people that have similar interests, such as hiking, biking, and knitting, or people in the same age group. This tool can be extremely helpful for those sitting at home wondering how and where to make new friends. Additionally, social media sites like *www.Facebook.com* can be helpful tools when used properly. A recent study in the *Journal of Abnormal Child Psychology* found that using social media for social comparison and feedback-seeking resulted in depressive symptoms and other cognitive impairments. The more the students in the study used social media networks, including Instagram and Facebook, the more depressive symptoms they exhibited.

Social networks and the Internet in general can provide a boost of feel-good chemicals in the short term, but can turn into dependency and addictive-type behavior. For the goal of optimal brain performance, these factors must be taken into consideration when creating a healthy lifestyle.

ESSENTIAL

Technology saves lives and has given modern civilization luxuries that would have been unfathomable even a hundred years ago. A balance of "screen time" and real life experiences is best. Not only does getting outdoors and away from screens boost your mood with vitamin D absorption and serotonin production, but it strengthens your eye muscles to look afar, possibly reducing your need for supplemental vision devices (contacts and glasses).

Sleep Tight for Brain Health

Insufficient quantity or quality of sleep is a stressor to the body. Sleep is a process that is essential to human health. Even though you may lie in bed for eight hours, that doesn't mean you get the benefits of eight hours of sleep.

The simple truth is that as a human, you are designed to wake up with the sun and go to bed with the sun. Granted, that doesn't mean you have to go to bed at 5 P.M. during the winter. That would be nearly impossible for most. However, staying up until midnight or later (unless required by your profession) is not the best choice. The evening hours are when melatonin, a sleep hormone that fights cancer, rises to its highest level with the intention of nourishing and protecting your mind and body. The active sleeping and dreaming processes allow your mind to determine what is important and what is not. One could think of dreaming as a filtering process to weed out irrelevant sights and sounds experienced during waking hours.

FACT

Sleep is not optional, nor is it a luxury. Sleep is a requirement for the healthy regulation of hormonal processes, detoxification, and immeasurable other functions. A healthy, focused, and active person during the day is one who sleeps and recovers with equal dedication. When sleep deficits occur, you can expect your memory, attention, and overall mood to slump as well.

You may have stayed up too late one night to discover that the next day you could not focus, maintain your attention, or maybe even your consciousness. Maintaining a regular sleep schedule is a key foundation to a healthy diet that will result in improved brain performance, focus, attention, mental clarity, and all other positive effects you are seeking. A realistic bedtime for the average 9-to-5 worker is the lights out at 10 P.M., with cell phones and all other sources of light out of the bedroom. Your bedroom should be a place for sleep and sex only, to properly program the brain to expect only these actions while you're there. Playing on your phone or computer in bed teaches the brain that it should be awake and producing energy to help you stay on task instead of sleeping. If you find that noise keeps you awake, a white noise machine can be helpful.

CHAPTER 2

Your Brain Chemicals Run the Show

Brain chemicals called neurotransmitters control many of your moods, emotions, and other sensations. Scientists have identified over 100 of them, and more continue to be discovered. Whether you are experiencing a blissful moment, a period of sadness, or seasonal depression, the basic underlying mechanism of action relies on a healthy balance of these brain chemicals. Without a proper balance of neurotransmitters, one can crave anything from sugar and alcohol to cigarettes and violent television. Achieving balance is the key to success and health.

What Are Neurotransmitters?

Neurotransmitters are brain chemicals that are responsible for many different conscious and subconscious reactions in the mind and body. Although scientists, neuroscientists, and other researchers have found over 100 different neurotransmitters, there are six commonly discussed neurotransmitters that play a huge role in your daily life and that determine the way you feel and act.

ESSENTIAL

When you feel confident and capable of handling stress, thank your neurotransmitters. When you feel anxious, blame your neurotransmitters. You may just need a walk in the woods or a supplemental form of the calming neurotransmitter, GABA, to relax your nervous system and allow you to enjoy your flight from Los Angeles to New York City without issue.

There are two kinds of neurotransmitters, inhibitory and excitatory. One is not better than the other; they need to be in balance to keep your system functioning properly and give you a healthy and stable mood. People who do not have a balance of neurotransmitters are likely to suffer from cravings, mood disorders, weight issues, poor concentration, and a generally suboptimal performance. While the world of brain chemicals can be extremely complex, the goal of this chapter is to give a basic overview of what neurotransmitters are, the causes and effects of altered neurotransmitter levels, and how these chemicals play a role in optimizing your mental, physical, and overall performance.

Excitatory Neurotransmitters

Excitatory neurotransmitters help keep you moving. Dopamine, norepinephrine, and epinephrine are three of the most powerful brain chemicals that are responsible for focus, drive, memory, and the general ability to handle what life throws at you. Coffee, caffeine, cigarettes, sugar, and other forms of stimulants directly impact the amount of dopamine produced in your brain. It's easy to become a victim to your own brain chemicals if you do not maintain a healthy balance. Dopamine will be discussed in greater detail shortly, but for now understand that addictive behavior and the "chasing the dragon" phenomena are tightly linked with this brain chemical.

Epinephrine (Adrenaline)

You are highly in touch with the effects of epinephrine and norepinephrine, even though you may not have heard these terms before. (You can use the terms adrenaline and noradrenaline interchangeably, depending on what is easier for you to understand.) These two excitatory neurotransmitters have similar and differential effects on the mind and body. Epinephrine, or adrenaline, is a key component of many first-aid kits. It is an essential emergency chemical for those with severe allergies who may suffer allergic reactions that can severely impact the normal functioning of breathing pathways and more. Many people are familiar with the EpiPen, a medical device for injecting epinephrine (adrenaline) into the body. People who are at risk of suffering anaphylactic shock typically carry an EpiPen near their person. These devices contain a specific amount of epinephrine—only enough to deliver one potentially life-saving dose.

Norepinephrine

Norepinephrine acts as both a neurotransmitter and a hormone. When under significant stress, norepinephrine causes an increase in blood sugar and heart rate to ensure adequate fuel to deal with or escape a threat. If you recall the discussion about modern civilization, you'll remember that daily stressors can influence brain chemicals. Rush-hour traffic, e-mails, and intimidating bosses can all contribute to your nervous system cranking itself up to respond.

Your nervous system relies on many chemicals, but the ones that you feel the most are these excitatory neurotransmitters. The shakiness and nervousness in your hands, the rapid heart rate and breathing, and the feelings of heaviness or lightness can all be attributed to the rise and release of excitatory neurotransmitters. This is normal. Humans would have not made it to the top of the food chain if they were not able to "rise to the occasion" when it was time to hunt, fight, or defend against other humans or predators. This ancient system has been hijacked by the incessant stress of the modern world that creates the feelings of impending doom, distorted time perception, and fear.

Remember that time you had to stand up in front of your peers and present something? Although your life was never in danger, it sure felt like it! Your general unsteadiness, sweaty palms, and fear of the unknown took hold on your ability to focus. You may have even completely forgotten what you were supposed to talk about. The brain doesn't have time to care about thinking clearly; it just wants to run away from the danger so that you can survive. In this instance, the body is tricked . . . there isn't a tiger in the room after all—it's just your boss or your teacher.

Learning how to control your nervous system can make or break your success in these types of situations. Even if you don't frequently engage in public speaking or other types of stressful events that put you in the spotlight, it's a good idea to be prepared. In those moments where seconds feel like minutes, keeping your nervous system under at least partial control will allow you to do that.

The Most Common Neurotransmitters

The average person knows serotonin as the "happiness chemical," but there are some forgotten neurotransmitters that play an equally important role in your ability to focus, perform, and relax. With an imbalance or deficiency of any or all of these common neurotransmitters, you could experience anxiety, burnout, brain fog, lethargy, and generally feel subpar. Optimizing them is an easy and realistic task that will greatly benefit your daily life.

Serotonin

Serotonin is likely the most well-known and discussed neurotransmitter. In the past couple of decades, it has become a household term. However, most people don't fully understand how this important brain chemical works, and don't realize the importance of maintaining a healthy balance of serotonin with the other neurotransmitters. Just because a little bit of something is good doesn't automatically mean that more of the same thing is better. This is especially the case with serotonin. It is true that serotonin plays a role in depression and mood disorders, but it is not always the root cause of the issue; assuming that you need drugs to fix you because you have a couple of bad days in a row isn't always necessary.

Research by Dr. Doeyoung Kim, MD and Michael Camilleri, MD published in the *American Journal of Gastroenterology* has found that the brain is not the primary location for serotonin; it has been estimated that about

95 percent of serotonin is found in the gastrointestinal tract. This is a huge breakthrough and quite a positive finding, because it reduces some of the complexity of optimizing serotonin levels naturally. Instead of immediately targeting the brain, looking downward into the gut (sometimes referred to as the "second brain") can hold significant potential for improving your mood and cognition.

Serotonin is thought to play a role in:

- Mood and behavior
- Appetite and relationship with food
- Sleep quality
- Sexual desire and function

Serotonin is not the only player when dealing with cognitive impairment such as depression. If it were that simple, the estimated one in ten people taking the antidepressant drugs known as SSRIs should feel better. But a study from the *New England Journal of Medicine* reported that over 30 percent of the FDA-registered studies on antidepressant agents were never published. Thirty-seven out of thirty-eight positive studies were published, but studies viewed by the FDA as having negative or questionable results were, with three exceptions, either not published or published in a way that conveyed a positive outcome. This selective reporting of clinical trial results can have adverse consequences for researchers, study participants, healthcare professionals, and patients because a clear representation of the poor effectiveness of these drugs is not revealed.

Dr. Mark Hyman wrote an article for the *Huffington Post* titled, "Why Antidepressants Don't Work for Treating Depression," which outlines the fact that 80 percent of people get better with just a placebo pill. So the saying "it's all in your head" might be right. Dr. Eric Braverman, the former chief clinical researcher at the Princeton Brain Bio Center, has appeared on numerous national radio and television programs from *Larry King Live* to *The David Letterman Show* and is a world-leading expert in the field of neurotransmitters. Braverman has written one of the best books on the topic of cognitive enhancement in the relationship between sub-optimal neurotransmitter levels. The book, called *The Edge Effect*, goes into great detail about the symptoms of various neurotransmitter deficiencies. Since deficiencies are so widespread, this book focuses on actionable steps.

However, Dr. Braverman's website *http://pathmed.com* has a free brain deficiency quiz that can be helpful for gaining a better understanding of your brain chemicals. On the topic of serotonin, he suggests that someone with low serotonin has the following symptoms:

- Sleep issues
- Doesn't feel like exercising
- Can't relax
- Night sweats
- Wakes up at least two times per night
- Difficulty falling back asleep once awakened
- Is sad
- Craves salt

It is said that minor to moderate deficiencies can be treated without medications, usually responding to a combination of natural/nutritional supplements and lifestyle changes. You will later learn about available brain-boosting compounds that can make the difference between you going through life with your head down and you prancing, dancing, and singing down the street.

ESSENTIAL

Brain chemistry changes by the second. Humans alter neurotransmitters with doughnuts, cookies, soda, and caffeine on a daily basis without understanding the underlying changes they are creating. Every action, thought, and especially food-like drug alters neurotransmitter levels, which results in a mood-altering effect. It's important to remove or reduce these neurotransmitter-altering compounds, because they cause more harm than good. Excess stress, anger, and a fast-paced life cause the same. Take time out for yourself if you want to feel your best.

Dopamine

As previously mentioned, dopamine is a neurotransmitter linked to pleasure, reward, drive, and personal motivation. People who have low dopamine levels may have trouble getting off of the couch and are reluctant to engage in activity. Those who have low activity levels but engage in dopamine-boosting behavior (such as smoking cigarettes, playing video games, watching violent or sexual content, or otherwise "risky behavior" activities) are artificially activating the brain's reward system.

Through an evolutionary lens, dopamine would have given early humans the motivation, dedication, and pleasure in the act of hunting and gathering food to provide for themselves and their family. In this context, living a stagnant life would have meant death. You could assume that the most successful hunting and gathering cultures had adequate levels of dopamine to get the tasks necessary for surviving and thriving completed.

In the modern world, people continue to exist with low dopamine levels and still survive since they don't have to directly hunt or forage for food. Where motivation and personal drive wane, delivery services and drive-through restaurants pick up the slack. Convenience is not necessarily a bad thing, but it can prevent you from creating and nourishing a healthy brain. Making a concerted effort to maintain healthy levels of brain chemicals is easier than you think.

FACT

In the medical field, dopamine is primarily only discussed in the instance of Parkinson's disease, where extremely low levels of dopamine are exhibited. There are some benefits to supporting the natural production of dopamine levels with supplements and other medications, but the disease is far more powerful then the current level of treatment available.

Deciphering the Dopaminergic System

The reason that cigarettes and other addictions are so hard to break is due to the dopaminergic system. After smoking or engaging in behavior that boosts dopamine levels for an extended period of time, pathways in the brain get "carved," which creates an even stronger addiction. The brain then realizes that all it has to do to get a hint of dopamine is to engage in the same behavior that gave the hit of dopamine last time. It's a vicious cycle that can actually be used to your benefit. Exercise can be a natural and healthful way of boosting dopamine levels. Some people take it to the extreme and have what's called "exercise addiction," where they feel depleted or depressed if they take a day off from the gym. As continually alluded to, a healthy balance of action and inaction is key.

FACT

The "pulling effect" that social media, e-mail, and other networks have to suck you in are based on the dopamine system. It's no wonder that people will get on their phones as soon as they wake up; it stimulates dopamine production, which helps them get out of bed. There are better ways to stimulate dopamine production, such as getting exposure to natural, bright light.

If you have adequate dopamine levels, your personality will be characterized by plenty of motivation, willpower, physical energy, and focus on the task at hand. You will wake up ready to face the day and whatever challenges you may encounter. Getting out of bed will seem as simple as brushing your teeth, not requiring much energy or emotional input. You will have the stamina to get through your day without craving sugar, caffeine, or refined carbohydrates and processed foods that will give you a short-lived boost.

Acetylcholine

Like most neurotransmitters, acetylcholine plays a role in both the nervous system and the physical body. Acetylcholine was the first neurotransmitter to be identified by Henry Hallett Dale in 1914 for its role in healthy heart function. Acetylcholine is derived from choline, a micronutrient naturally found in many foods. If you need more reason to eat healthy, organic eggs, the abundance of choline in egg yolks supports healthy acetylcholine levels. This type of fat is also found in grass-fed beef and fish, and is incredibly helpful for supporting optimal brain function.

Choline consumption isn't just healthy for adults; human breast milk contains great amounts of choline, since it is necessary for the proper development of a newborn's brain and liver. In fact, the choline content of human breast milk doubles six to seven days after birth, making it a much more complete nutritional source than formula for the baby. This is another reason and example of how Mother Nature got it right.

Acetylcholine plays an important role in both memory and learning. Neurodegenerative disease is often found when acetylcholine levels are extremely low. The link between Alzheimer's disease and acetylcholine is strong. Alzheimer's disease is a serious brain disorder in which levels of acetylcholine can drop by up to 90 percent. The continual death of brain cells is what causes significant loss of cognitive function, memory, and other normal behavior functions. The memory center of the brain, the hippocampus, is unable to perform its duties of converting and storing short-term memory to long-term memory, which causes forgetfulness of present and past experiences. People who forget where they put their keys or why they entered a room may be suffering from some level of acetylcholine deficiency. Similar to Parkinson's disease, Alzheimer's disease has no cure, but nutritional supplementation has shown some benefit. A deeper understanding of the impact of brain chemical deficiencies throughout life must be researched.

GABA

GABA (gamma-aminobutyric acid) is a chemical produced in the brain that is far less common than the aforementioned neurotransmitters. You can think of GABA as the "brakes of the brain," since it is commonly recommended as an over-the-counter supplement for anti-anxiety and relaxing effects. Adequate levels of GABA are what allow you to feel calm and satiated when you eat. GABA has been shown to improve many brain functions, such as memory and study capability. GABA allows you to handle stressful situations without excessive nervous tension or anxiety.

ESSENTIAL

GABA levels and your ability to relax are determined by genetics, foods, lifestyle, and other factors. If you are someone who is always wound tight, pay close attention to the supplemental methods you can use to restore healthy GABA levels. Responding calmly to a serious situation may save your life one day.

Caffeine, the world's main drug of choice, depletes GABA levels. This is why people who drink coffee may also suffer from anxiety, irritability, panic attacks, and general nervous tension. Drinking alcohol temporarily boosts

GABA levels, which is part of the reason why alcohol is so popular at social events. The significant boost in serotonin levels combined with a moderate boost in GABA levels creates a one-two punch effect for reducing social anxiety and generally making the current situation feel a bit smoother. When these two neurotransmitter levels are altered and fluctuate after the consumption of alcohol, cognitive function and the ability to think rationally are affected.

Anti-anxiety medications commonly target the GABA receptors in the brain and are very effective at reducing the instance of panic attacks, shortness of breath, and other generally benign symptoms of low GABA levels. However, these drugs don't regulate the brain's ability to produce GABA, leading to dependence, withdrawal, and potentially worse anxiety than the level that led the person to begin taking anti-anxiety drugs in the first place. This goes to show how important the safe modification of levels of brain chemicals must be.

ALERT

The GABA molecule is supposed to be too big to give a relaxing effect in those that consume it via supplementation. If a person has a condition similar to leaky gut, called "leaky brain," these larger molecules and other toxins can slip through and give the desired relaxing effect. This isn't necessarily a good thing. You want a solid blood brain barrier. Removing gluten and other inflammatory compounds from the diet can begin the healing and sealing process of both of these barriers.

Stimulants can be useful for boosting energy and productivity, but when taken in excess, you can surpass the balancing capacity of GABA, leading to diminished cognitive performance. In other words, one cup of coffee may make you feel great and turn on your brain, allowing you to focus, multitask, and take care of what you need to do. Drinking two cups of coffee or more may make you feel foggy, tired, and generally inefficient overall. You may even experience nervous tension, shaky hands, or anxiety.

For starters, meditation is a simple and effective way of boosting GABA levels. Some consider yoga as a form of moving meditation, and the perceived high at the end of the session can be directly attributed to a boost in both endorphins and GABA levels. Next time you are stressed, spend a few minutes focusing on your breath to naturally boost your GABA levels and prevent you from having a stress-induced catastrophe either mentally or physically. Cultivating a relaxation practice such as meditating, doing yoga, or walking in nature can be a great way to support a balanced and relaxed brain.

Epinephrine and Norepinephrine

Also known as adrenaline and noradrenaline, these two neurotransmitters can be lumped together since they both play major roles in the sympathetic nervous system and stress response. Adrenaline is secreted by the adrenal glands, two walnut-sized glands that sit on top of your kidneys. The inner region of the adrenal gland is called the medulla. The medulla produces adrenaline, noradrenaline, and dopamine.

Without your adrenal glands, you couldn't survive. A rare autoimmune disease known as Addison's disease only entered the mainstream conversation when it was revealed that President John Kennedy was suffering from it. This disease essentially kills the adrenal glands and curtails your ability to withstand any amount of stress, causing you to become dizzy, fatigued, and stricken with weakness and weight loss.

Healthy adrenal glands are essential in dealing with and adapting to a changing world. Later in this book you will learn how a category of compounds called *adaptogens* can be used to safely and successfully support your stress response and nervous system. You may be able to go from a nervous wreck to a strong-willed warrior with the help of these compounds. Developing a stress response toolkit for both daily and acute use will be one of the most helpful strategies you can implement to overcome life's challenges.

Adrenaline is unique in the fact that it acts as both a hormone and neurotransmitter. This means that it can alter both your mental and physical abilities. In the medical field, adrenaline is used to treat heart attacks or other issues relating to the heart.

In terms of evolution, adrenaline would have been necessary to perform the intense tasks of sprinting, catching, and hunting prey. Production of adrenaline and other hormones such as cortisol rise in stressful situations to allow increased brain function and physical performance. When a tiger comes out of the jungle and ends up face-to-face with you and your family, adrenaline and cortisol initiate the fight-or-flight response. At certain times in evolutionary history, fleeing would have made more sense than fighting, and vice versa. Today, fighting or fleeing may not be necessary at all; rather, a rational and calm conversation to sort out a disagreement might be what's required. This is hard to do for some people, because the fight-or-flight system is genetically hardwired more deeply then the more recent ability to think rationally and solve problems with the mind.

Balance Is Key

It cannot be overstated that balance is key for a healthy and optimal functioning brain. Just because you can take a supplement that is geared for boosting one brain chemical doesn't mean that you should take more of it, or take it for a longer duration. There are complex feedback loops that should be handled lightly and adjusted on a cyclical basis.

To keep it simple, if coffee is making you feel anxious and you can't seem to focus even after drinking it, try removing it. If you find the only thing that gives you pleasure is to consume sugar, go for a walk instead the next time you have a craving.

Humans are more than capable of naturally supporting healthy brain function, and should be healthy and happy as a default. It's when the system is hijacked by modern conveniences such as artificial sweeteners, refined sugars, processed foods, television, and other recent inventions when you forget what normal is supposed to feel like, and how you are supposed to attain this so-called normal mood.

Changing your health is essential for reaching optimal brain performance. This is not a restricting and miserable experience, as portrayed by diet companies who convince you that you can still be healthy and eat your brownies, just as long as you don't eat too many of them. Creating a lifestyle and nutritional regimen that nourishes the brain can be more enjoyable and pleasurable then you have imagined.

Remember that you are a unique individual, and that your results when altering your neurotransmitter levels will vary. Just because your spouse can consume coffee and does quite well with it doesn't mean that you will. You may find that coffee makes you feel anxious and shaky. You could have lower levels of the calming chemical, GABA, in your brain than he or she does. This isn't a life sentence of anxiety or other potentially uncomfortable emotions; simply a learning process that will allow you to successfully transition yourself into the person who you want to be, feeling how you want to feel. There is hope for upgrading your mental performance.

CHAPTER 3

Healthy Habits for a Healthy Brain

Take a deep breath. You may feel overwhelmed or even stressed about the task of safely managing your moods and improving your cognitive performance. Rest assured that although all this information about neurotransmitters can feel intimidating, there are many simple strategies to apply to your diet and lifestyle that can significantly impact and improve your ability to focus, feel, and enjoy life. There are roadblocks and hurdles that will attempt to block your path to health, but you'll soon rid them from your sights.

The Food-Mood Connection

If you've purchased this book, it's likely that you have a basic knowledge of the importance of healthy food choices, not only for your physical health (in the case of building muscle or losing weight), but also in the knowledge that what you eat directly impacts the way you feel, think, and function.

Each bite you take either helps or hurts your ability to focus clearly, make decisions, and drive creativity. The choices you make on a daily basis are not benign. This is a good thing. You are able to significantly shift your mindset and alter the course of your genetic susceptibility through these choices. The field of epigenetics has proven that you are not bound by the constraints of your cognitive ability that may have been passed down from your parents or further along the ancestral line.

The food-mood connection is best described by looking at your hunter-gatherer ancestors. The foods your ancestors ate would have always been natural and organic, and there would have been no need to distinguish between a healthy food and a non-healthy food. Calorie counting and reading the ingredient label were not a thing. Mother Nature herself would have regulated the foods available.

Visualize the place you live in the wintertime. What foods are available? Do the foods you eat match the foods that are locally available?

Sugar's Impact

Hunter-gatherers loved sugar too, and would gorge on honey and fruit when the time was right. However, it was generally an infrequent and special occasion that honey was extracted from beehives. It would have been a celebratory event where the tribe gathered and licked their fingers in unison. There are a number of biological processes that normally regulate the ability to deal with the intake of these sugars that are simply overburdened in the modern world.

FACT

Sugar is one of the most highly abused drugs in the world due to its ability to boost your mood. It boosts neurotransmitters temporarily, but the effect on the pancreas is far worse than the benefit. The blood sugar rollercoaster exhausts the organs of the ability to regulate blood sugar, causing your energy and mood to subsequently slump.

When sugar is consumed, the hormone insulin must rise to store the sugar away. It is an emergency situation if too much sugar remains in the bloodstream. A great place for the body to store excess sugar, or glucose, is in the fat cells. A reasonable amount of fat on the skeletal system is necessary and healthful to protect the organs from damage and extreme temperatures. However, excess visceral fat is not only harmful for the function of the physical body, but impairs cognitive ability as well.

Excess sugars, which include not only standard table sugar but excess carbohydrates such as bread and pasta, cause a process called *glycation*. This process creates something known as advanced glycation end products, or AGE. There couldn't be a better acronym, because these enzymes essentially age you. These substances age not only the physical body, but the brain as well, and are linked to neurodegeneration in the form of Alzheimer's disease. In fact, Dr. Mark Hyman refers to Alzheimer's disease as "type 3 diabetes." *The Journal of Alzheimer's Disease* has proposed this term since Alzheimer's represents a neuro-endocrine disorder that resembles (yet is distinct from) diabetes. Cognitive impairment is directly linked to the consumption of refined carbohydrates and forms of sugar. There is a reason that other cultures don't age as quickly as those in the developed world. There is a genetic component, but there is also a general lack of refined sugars and convenient foods that are abundant in the developed world.

ESSENTIAL

If you are struggling with sugar addiction, a particular amino acid called L-Glutamine can be very helpful at squelching the urge to eat a cookie when you're feeling tired and moody. It acts as a quick fuel source for the brain to keep working optimally. Don't skip meals either, because it can cause rash decisions that you may regret!

Use Food As Medicine

You can't produce healthy and happy chemicals out of thin air. You must obtain the raw materials, or building blocks, necessary to create them. A low-protein diet impairs the ability to manufacture such chemicals.

Under times of stress, the most appealing food choice may be sugar, candy, chocolate, wine, or another quick fix. While these choices may create a quick burst of brain chemicals to make you feel good, you could end up more depleted than before. Sugar is a stressor to the body that depletes the stores of vitamins and minerals.

Instead, making a bowl of guacamole and eating organic blue corn chips could be a far more satiating option for your belly and your brain. Some may laugh at this food swap, but after you consistently consume healthy fats and proteins during times of stress and food cravings, you'll realize how effective they can be! It's a quite empowering experience to be in charge of what you eat.

Quality over Quantity

You'd be surprised how full and happy you can be while eating less. Society tends to classify people into two categories: those that gorge themselves and those that starve themselves for the supposed benefits. But what if you could just eat until you are satisfied?

Okinawa, Japan has the highest concentration of centenarians in the world. These 100-plus-year-olds also have the lowest occurrence of heart disease, stroke, and cancer in the world. Their secret lies in many dietary habits, including the fact that the importance of food quality is encouraged in their culture. An even more specific habit they follow is that of *hara hachi bu*, which translates to eating only until 80 percent full.

Of course, this doesn't mean that consuming honey buns and soft drinks until you are 80 percent full will create health and happiness beyond that initial moment. Okinawans still focus on nutrient-dense food choices such as sweet potatoes and fermented foods, which supply beneficial bacteria to nourish the gut where serotonin is manufactured.

Is it any surprise that the people who have some of the most nutrient-dense diets in the world are the happiest and longest-lived? They are reducing the amount of oxidative stress in their diet and seem to live a lifestyle that moves a little slower than the rest of the world. Maybe the goals of more productivity, squeezing every ounce out of each day, and total world domination should be reconsidered.

Stabilize Your Blood Sugar

Blood sugar is a topic that only diabetics generally care about. They have to care, because it's key to their survival. However, it's important to the otherwise healthy individual as well, because of the link between blood sugar dysfunction and mood disorders. If you intend to have a steady, focused mind, you must have a similar structure to your blood sugar.

The blood-sugar rollercoaster that most Americans are on is quite detrimental to cognitive performance. For example, starting the day with coffee and sugar will boost up brain chemicals and the blood sugar level together. It will make the person feel energetic and maybe even happy for a short time. But by the time 10 A.M. rolls around, this person is exhausted, grumpy, and hungry. The slang term "hangry," or hungry and angry, is accurate. A blood sugar level that crashes after this intake of carbs and/or sugar will cause mood instability, brain fog, and concentration loss until the blood sugar has stabilized once again. Some people will also suffer headaches and a general spacey feeling from a lack of stabilized blood sugar.

Juicing and Blood Sugar

While there are great benefits in juicing, or extracting the nutrients from fruits and vegetables, it is a common practice than can act as a roadblock in stabilizing the blood sugar of an individual. When you juice a fruit or vegetable, you are left with only the raw materials of nutrients, minerals, and natural sugar content. This isn't bad for you; it just isn't the optimal way to consume your fruits and vegetables. By juicing, you remove the fiber component of the fruit that allows for a slow release of the natural sugar content into the bloodstream. Remove this buffering mechanism and you are essentially taking a shot of nutrient-rich sugar. Once again, it isn't inherently bad for you, it's just not the best way to get your nutrients.

If you are in such a rush that you can't sit down to eat your fruits and vegetables, make a smoothie. Instead of separating the fruit from the fiber, you use the entire edible portion of the fruit allowing you to process the sugar at a much slower rate. This may result in more satiety and longer-lasting energy overall. Adding a protein and fat source to your smoothie, such as grass-fed whey protein and coconut oil, can take your nutrient density from average to exceptional. Since your brain is primarily composed of fat, it needs adequate levels of fat for fuel, and more importantly, cognitive performance!

A Brain-Healthy Diet

While this isn't a diet book per se, sticking a list of some of the dietary foundations on your refrigerator can be one of the most helpful and important steps. In fact, optimizing your diet is by far the most powerful and long-lasting modality for improving brain function available. No drug or other synthetic material will exceed the nutrient density found in plants, animals, herbs, and other natural foods and medicines. Do not underestimate the brain boosters that can be found at your local farmers' market or supermarket!

The Dietary Essentials

The following foods are key to a brain-healthy diet. When you are looking to boost your brainpower, consider including these foods in your daily diet.

Grass-Fed and Organic Meats

Many healthy humans eat meat. There are various amino acids and other naturally occurring constituents that act as precursors to neurotransmitters that fuel the brain and heart, such as taurine and tryptophan, found in meat. Dr. Weston A. Price, world explorer and dentist, did not find a single fully healthy vegetarian culture. There are many components necessary to healthy development and brain function found if you include this food group in your diet.

The steak at your chain restaurant will not be sufficient. They are usually conventionally raised meats that are fed genetically modified corn. When you see a new study come out about the dangers of red meat, remember that they are not using organic, grass-fed and pasture-raised, healthy, happy animals. Eating sick animals will make you sick.

Whenever possible, seek out, purchase, and consume grass-fed and organic meats on a weekly basis. Whether you prefer beef, bison, lamb, pork, or other type of meat, the quality is what counts. You don't have to stuff yourself with pounds and pounds of meat per week to be healthy. Even the healthiest of meats should not be over-consumed. Stick to a palm-sized portion of meat with each meal. You can find quality meat using the websites *www.localharvest.org* and *www.eatwild.com*.

Organic Vegetables and Fruits

Are any vegetables better than no vegetables? It depends who you ask. If you are consuming any of the fruits or vegetables that make up the Dirty Dozen (produce most contaminated by pesticide use, as rated by the Environmental Working Group), you may be taking on more risk than it's worth. The full list includes: apples, peaches, nectarines, strawberries, grapes, celery, spinach, sweet bell peppers, cucumbers, cherry tomatoes, imported snap peas, potatoes, hot peppers, kale, and collard greens.

ALERT

Pesticides are ubiquitous in conventional, or non-organic, food. According to the EWG executive summary, nearly two thirds of the 3,015 produce samples tested by the U.S. Department of Agriculture in 2013 contained pesticide residues. EWG investigates produce with the highest pesticide loads for their list known as the Dirty Dozen.

They found that 99 percent of apples, 98 percent of peaches, and 97 percent of nectarines tested positive for at least one pesticide residue. A single grape and sweet bell pepper sample contained 15 pesticides. Single samples of cherry tomatoes, nectarines, peaches, imported snap peas, and strawberries showed 13 different pesticides apiece.

Purchasing organic food is one of the best ways to protect yourself against these harmful chemicals that sabotage your cognitive ability and overall health. Even better, and sometimes cheaper, is to grow your own organic produce at home. If you live in an apartment or condo, you can easily grow herbs on a windowsill. Indoor plants help clean the air, which will also reduce your overall toxic load and support your cognitive function.

Organic Nuts and Seeds

Nature can be funny sometimes. Have you looked closely at a walnut? It looks very similar to a human brain, and happens to be one of the most nutrient-dense nuts. This nut will help nourish your brain and will provide the raw materials necessary to make neurotransmitters.

Since high-risk behaviors (including an unhealthy diet, lack of exercise, smoking, and exposure to environmental toxins) lead to oxidative stress, inflammation, and brain degeneration over a long period of time, it can be hard to track the benefits of seemingly simple food swaps such as a handful of walnuts instead of a typical sugary snack. But the *American Journal of Nutrition* states that walnuts are rich in numerous phytochemicals, including high amounts of polyunsaturated fatty acids, and offer potential benefits to brain health. Polyphenolic compounds found in walnuts reduce the oxidant inflammatory load on brain cells and improve brain signaling. It was also found that walnuts increase neurogenesis, the growth of new brain cells.

There is no such thing as consuming pesticides in moderation. While it's a little bit harder to find organic nuts and seeds than produce, it's an equally important distinction to make when stocking a brain-boosting pantry. If cognitive performance and weight loss are your goals, nuts and seeds can be a great way to achieve it. Some of the best are pumpkin seeds, walnuts, almonds, cashews, macadamias, pecans, and Brazil nuts. Those sugar-coated, chocolate-covered, and roasted ones you find at the carnival, unfortunately, don't count.

Healthy Fats

Butter was a popular food item up until around World War II when the development of hydrogenated fats and oils was necessary to provide a longer shelf life for foods that were transported around the world for soldiers.

Butter continued to fall out of favor as the low-fat era began decades after the war ended. Low-fat diets were incredibly popular. It took several more decades for failed dieters and scientists to come to the same consensus: Dietary fat is a healthful and necessary component of a human's life. Without it, your nervous system and metabolism aren't able to function normally, and the body holds on to fat as a protective mechanism. If there is no fat being consumed in the diet, the body determines that there must be a famine present . . . and holds on to all the fat it can to ensure survival.

On the opposite end of the spectrum, you have moderate and high-fat diets that have helped people lose hundreds of pounds without starving or counting calories. Forgetting that fat is one of the most prized components of an animal to indigenous peoples has contributed to the obesity epidemic. Adding healthy fats to your diet can make the difference between a suffering, obese, and depressed human and a happy, lean, and energetic one.

The best sources of healthy fats are:

- Organic coconut oil
- Grass-fed butter
- Ghee, or clarified butter
- Pastured fats from pork, chicken, lamb, duck and beef
- Olive oil
- Avocado oil
- Sesame oil
- Walnut oil

As you may have noticed, "fake fats" and other oils such as margarine, canola oil, corn oil, vegetable oil, soybean oil, grapeseed oil, sunflower oil, safflower oil, Crisco, and the like are all excluded. These are highly processed oils that are likely undergoing oxidation and are on the way to rancidity by the time you consume them.

ESSENTIAL

A good starting place for finding a healthy eating tribe in your local area is to search and join a local chapter of the Weston A. Price Foundation. You can mingle with others who seek optimal health and happiness, share recipes, and even find the best source for your organic meats, produce, and butter at these events.

Including healthy fats in your diet will not only jump-start your weight loss and help you lose those few extra pounds, but it will fuel your brain more efficiently and longer than ever before. Just like a car runs best on race fuel, your brain runs best on healthy fats. Use organic fats liberally on top of your meals or to cook with.

Brain-Busters to Avoid

So far you have learned about the importance of choosing organic produce, meats, nuts, and fats, but there are several other brain-busters that can make the difference between having a brain like a dazed zombie or an accurate, precise, and healthy one.

The following should be avoided when brain health is the goal:

- Inflammatory oils
- Sugar and refined carbohydrates, such as boxed meals, breads, pastas, bagels, and anything else that didn't come directly from the earth, a tree, an animal, a bush, etc.
- Caffeine in excess

There are dozens, if not hundreds, of perpetrators attempting to directly or indirectly sabotage your brain health and mental performance. Focus on what you can control and remove as many stressors from your diet and life as possible. At some point, the stress of stressing will override the benefits of your healthy diet. Obsessiveness and starving yourself because something isn't 100 percent organic at a restaurant isn't well warranted.

Reduce Your Stress Load

It's helpful to look at your overall stress load as if it were a rain barrel. If you have a little bit of rain in your barrel, you will remain alive. If you have too much rain, you have a flood and have other consequences to clean up. If you have a little stress, that's good. You are alive. But if your "stress barrel" is overflowing, you're at risk for burnout, cognitive impairment, and other health issues. You don't have to avoid stress like the plague—you just have to develop a healthy balance between stress and relaxation.

Stress and the Brain

The memory center that is affected in neurodegenerative disease is the same one that is affected by chronic stress. After all, chronic stress in some form is at the root of nearly every ailment. The elevation and subsequent depletion of cortisol and other stress hormones causes depression, memory impairments, and other physical effects such as hair loss and slow wound-healing time. The brain and body take a hit in unison.

Stress is partially about perception. If you think you have too much stress, you probably do. But if you think you have a handle on your stress load, your mind and body adjust accordingly. Those memes and quotes posted across social media have some truth to them. Don't fear life; chase your dreams at full speed ahead. You can do it! This attitude is actually quite helpful in programming the brain to cope with stress in a healthier manner.

The other mindset, one of hopelessness, doubt, and fear, can be partially traced back to neurotransmitter deficiencies, but also come from your conscious thoughts. If you tell yourself (or others tell you) that you aren't capable of success and are destined to fail at life, your mind and body will accept defeat. Athletes and professionals attest to the importance of "faking it until you make it." If you aren't comfortable, keep your head up and accept the situation. While you may not be able to change the situation, you can change how you react to it.

Walk to Reduce Stress

Walking in nature and similar meditation practices are very important. These activities engage the parasympathetic nervous system and counteract the effects of the "go-go-go" lifestyle. It's safe to say that you and your peers need more parasympathetic time than the latter.

It's been shown that a 15-minute walk in nature can lower your cortisol levels by 12.4 percent. Parasympathetic activity is also enhanced by 55 percent, indicating a relaxed state of the nervous system. The goal is to proactively respond to life's stressors, as opposed to simply reacting. This capability is improved by making nature walks a regular habit.

Smart Supplementation

Different lifestyles require different amounts and types of nutrients. Taking a particular supplement just because you heard about it from an advertisement or website isn't always the most effective approach. Instead, learning about many different nutrients, minerals, herbs, and other compounds and what they do for you can be a much more targeted approach to safe and effective supplementation.

The facts are in: For optimal health, one must take supplements. Unless you are living in a part of the world that is free from air, water, and soil pollution, eat only 100 percent fresh, organically grown animals and plants, and are outside multiple hours per day getting exercise and sunlight, it's impossible to get all of the nutrients your mind and body need. Unfortunately, there are not considerable amounts of untarnished land free from human influence and pollution to escape to. This shouldn't discourage you, because it's entirely possible to have a great dietary foundation supported by a synergy of nutrients. Due to soil depletion and an indoor, generally sedentary lifestyle, it makes sense to add these nutrients back in the form of supplements such as vitamin D and magnesium.

You will learn about magnesium and vitamin D and their nootropic-like effects shortly, but for now, understand that your cabinet, pantry, refrigerator, freezer, and garden are all equally important. Where any of these places are found lacking, supplements can attempt to fill in the gaps. Supplements are designed to *supplement*, not replace any nutrient or other measure that can be obtained from diet or lifestyle.

Using Supplements to Adapt to Life's Changes

Life is always changing, and so is a good supplement regimen. For example, if you are under significant amounts of stress, you will need more than usual amounts of vitamin C, B vitamins, magnesium, and other minerals. The body is generally capable of handling periods of intense stress, but it does cause depletion of the nutrients, minerals, and other "fuel sources" necessary to keep the adrenal glands and nervous system operating at full capacity.

After a certain period of time, depending on factors such as diet, lifestyle, genetics, perception of stress, and more, you may burn out. This is characterized by freezing up during times of stress and not being able to act properly, or at all. When you once stood up and fought back and conquered your stressors, now you may be riddled with fear, anxiety, and/or general overwhelming feelings.

This is where nutrients such as adaptogenic herbs come into play. These compounds allow the body to gently but efficiently become more resilient to various types of stress, including hot or cold temperatures, mental or perceived stress, and physical stress. A single nutrient, or synergistic combination of multiple nutrients, essentially makes your "stress barrel" larger and causes it to fill up more slowly. You may be under the same stress that you were before you began taking these compounds, but dealing with it will seem more manageable.

CHAPTER 4

Classes of Nootropics

It is difficult to categorize supplements solely on the components they're made of. For example, the properties of one herb may sedate and relax you, while another property may boost your energy levels. The categories of nootropics discussed in this chapter are an attempt to organize and explain the various supplements, nutrients, and compounds based on their effects. From supplements that speed up the mind to those that give a gentle boost to your happiness and motivation levels, having a basic understanding of what you are trying to accomplish with these nootropics will determine which you choose.

The Neurotransmitter Buzzword

The reason that the world of nootropics has generated so much buzz in the past decade is not just because of the great potential for taking your lifestyle and cognitive ability into your own hands; it's also due to the fact that you can successfully modulate your brain chemistry with extreme specificity. There are various self-tests that can be found online that can help you discover neurotransmitter deficiencies. You can then determine a possible route of action and self-modification. Go to *www.notjustpaleo.com* for more information.

ALERT

Generally speaking, avoiding supplements in tablet form is a good idea, since they require potentially unhealthful fillers and binders to keep them molded together. Safe ingredients for tablets are now being created, but optimal absorption still may lack in those.

Neurotransmitter Testing

There is a lot of controversy surrounding the testing of neurotransmitters. Some argue that urine testing is an accurate way to find neurotransmitter deficiencies; this will determine what amino acids and nutrients are needed to correct the deficiencies. (This will also help you determine which nootropics you should take.) Others argue that a similar but different testing mechanism called the Organic Acids Test is more accurate and should be the standard for neurotransmitter testing. It is a simple urine test that is done from the comfort of your home. Instead of looking at the presence of specific nutrients in the blood, the OAT test looks for the effects of a nutrient deficiency by identifying byproducts that occur in the body when a deficiency exists. You can discover vitamin, mineral, and amino acid deficiencies on top of your antioxidant status, detoxification ability, neurotransmitter production and function, and more.

The Questionnaire Approach

A more holistic and simple approach to determining neurotransmitter deficiency was defined by Dr. Eric Braverman and Julia Ross, two of the world's leading neurotransmitter and neuro-nutrient therapy experts. In this method, readers fill out a questionnaire that outlines symptoms of each neurotransmitter deficiency. For example, if you have tense muscles and can't relax, you may have a GABA deficiency. There are supplement protocols given to target each deficiency. With a combined total of nearly 100 years of experience, their contributions to the field of neurotransmitter modification are derived from not just research and scientific papers, but experience from seeing and treating thousands of patients. They also teach others how to become practitioners, to use this simple assessment, and to properly understand and create treatment plans based on the results.

Choosing the Right Test for You

Just like a varied diet is the best approach to nutritional health, a varied approach to both neurotransmitter testing and experimentation makes sense for brain health. Some people need a piece of paper that gives them a clear diagnosis of their condition, while others might find success with the questionnaire approach.

Lab testing can be an extremely profitable business model for many practitioners, ranging from $100–$500 each. This doesn't mean you should avoid having neurotransmitter tests done; however, some people may not be financially capable of having these types of lab tests run. For those who may not be able to afford lab tests, or for those just beginning to explore this field, free online tests or questionnaires are the best ways to get started. Your own particular needs will determine the best route of action for testing.

Matches, Not Fire

Many in the media paint an image of smart drugs and dietary supplements as unsafe, dangerous, and like playing with fire. A more accurate analogy would be playing with matches—they aren't dangerous by themselves, but they require a fuel source, such as a pile of wood or even a building, to possess real potential danger.

While nutrients and supplements in general tend to be much more benign in terms of side effects and potential interactions, it's important to know that nutrients can be just as powerful as prescription drugs. This isn't said to instill fear, but to encourage respect and a level of understanding of what you are putting in your body. Some people aren't even aware that alcohol is a drug. It is so widely accepted in society and is available on nearly every street corner in the world that no one blinks an eye when they purchase a giant bottle of whiskey capable of causing death.

In general, supplements and nutrients do not cause death on their own, but they do interact with some of the same neurotransmitters that commonly used drugs (such as alcohol) also work on. The neurotransmitters serotonin and GABA are altered by both alcohol and many supplements. It's not necessarily dangerous to combine these two, but it's certainly not advised.

ALERT

Mixing prescription drugs or any other type of substance with supplements is not a wise decision. Unless you have a deep understanding of how these drugs work and which neurotransmitters are altered by both the drugs and the nutrients, or you have had clearance from a physician or other health care practitioner, take them at separate times of the day, if at all.

Organic Whenever Possible

Part of the reason that supplements are so powerful is because they absorb minerals and other compounds from the soil to create their therapeutic components. Just like fruits and vegetables, herbs and other earth-grown produce, supplements should be cultivated in an organic fashion whenever possible. This is not to say that supplements not grown in organic soil are ineffective or hold no value; it just isn't the optimal way to source ingredients.

If you are an athlete or someone who needs to perform at the top of your game in your work or personal life (which is nearly everyone), the attention to details are what separate the winners from the runners-up. If you are serious about your art or performance, choose organic ingredients whenever possible. It's not just for competition's sake, it's for the nourishment and protection of neurons—the brain cells that are allowing you to read and comprehend this material.

Ingredient Lab Testing

Most companies should publicly publish documents that verify the absence of heavy metals, mold, and other toxins that could be found in their products. If they do not have it listed on their website if applicable, you can call them and verify their purity.

Supplement impurities and contaminants are not a common issue because many supplement companies don't manufacture the products themselves anyway. They outsource manufacturing to one of many companies that take care of testing and any other necessary safety precautions.

You may have seen the lawsuit involving four companies—Walmart, Walgreens, GNC, and Target—that found themselves in hot water after it was announced that their store brands of herbal supplements didn't contain the promised amount of herbs. Four out of five products produced by these companies contained fillers and potentially hazardous materials to those with autoimmune conditions such as wheat and grass. Only 21 percent of store-brand herbal supplements contained the plants listed on the labels.

The phrase "you get what you pay for" could not be truer than in the supplement industry. Generally speaking, if a supplement you find is exponentially cheaper than that of a common or more reputable brand, dig deeper. They may be using a weaker extract of the material you are looking for, or they may just use less of that compound. Another tactic that saves money and provides a lower quality supplement is to use forms of nutrients that are not absorbed by the body.

For example, most mainstream brands use a form of magnesium called magnesium oxide in their mineral supplements. This form has been shown to have as low as a 4 percent absorption rate. More therapeutically focused companies use other forms of magnesium, such as magnesium glycinate or citrate, that have much higher absorption rates and therefore are more effective at giving the desired effect of the supplement.

Racetams

Racetams are a class of drugs that are designed to increase memory. Scientists do not have a clear understanding of how these drugs actually work. The mechanism of action is confusing simply because the brain is so complex and there are many different "knobs and widgets" that can be modified to give various effects, such as enhanced attention and improved focus and endurance for mental tasks. When using strict terminology, nootropics are referring to racetams. It's the other compounds and classes that may not fit the dictionary definition of a nootropic, but still have positive effects with minimal to no side effects.

What Are Racetams?

The racetam family of nootropics was developed in the 1960s and has since become a more widely used supplement. When people are referring to "smart drugs," they are typically referring to racetams. Most of them are generally mild and certainly will not create effects like those seen in Hollywood movies. You will not be able to digest the contents of an entire encyclopedia in one sitting, nor will you possess superpowers. The results you get from any supplement are determined from your starting point, tolerance, and unique biochemistry.

Racetams in particular are synthetic in nature, which raises a red flag for some people. They are capable of improving memory, cognitive performance, attention span, and other related markers. The funny thing is science still doesn't have a 100 percent clear picture on how these compounds work so well to create such benefits in the brain. The medical field has an idea that it has something to do with the glutamate receptors in the brain, which can change the efficiency of the brain. But since these substances are usually not prescription drugs, profit potential is low, resulting in a lack of interest in research studies.

This is why you must thoroughly investigate your options, and experiment accordingly. Some people may feel nothing after taking certain supplements, while others may feel incredible afterwards. Some may feel more tired than before they even took the supplement, while others may have an exponential positive impact on performance and productivity.

There are multiple categories and types of supplements listed throughout this book to allow you some room for contemplation and further research. Although clinical research is limited on certain compounds, various online forums and groups have formed to discuss their experiments in using them. Longecity.org is a great place to read stories and experiences with these nutrients.

Stacking

A term you may want to familiarize yourself with is *stacking*, which simply translates to taking multiple compounds, nutrients, herbs, etc. together to enhance the effects of one another. For example, some energy drinks may contain both vitamin B_{12} and vitamin B_6, which are both helpful in their own way at allowing you greater energy and motivation.

"Sleep stacks" may combine nutrients such as GABA and valerian root, a commonly recommended herb for insomnia and sleeplessness. GABA would be recommended to attempt and calm the nervous system, while valerian root would come into play to actually induce sleep. The term stacking is one you will find if and when you research further into the world of nootropics.

Start Slowly

It's always best to start with one nutrient or compound at a time so that you can accurately identify what is working for you and what is not. How can you successfully track your results if you begin taking five things at once? This is just a friendly reminder; some individuals like to go "all or nothing" and end up confused and broke! Supplements can become expensive, which is another good reason to try to find one that you like and that appears to be useful for your goals.

Adaptogens

Did the word "adapt" pop out at you upon reading the term adaptogen? It should have. This is a category of plants, herbs, nutrients, or other compounds that help the body adapt and overcome various forms of stress. Whether you are referring to physical stress in the form of exercise or you want increased cognitive performance and longevity, adaptogens are an extremely safe and effective class of substances that deserve the term nootropic.

Adaptogens range from medicinal mushrooms to herbs and roots. The different options offered by the plant kingdom are quite incredible. Adaptogens have been used for thousands of years, but actually naming the category of compounds that essentially switch on and off the stress modulators in the body didn't happen until the twentieth century. Adaptogens are said to decrease the reactivity of an organism, which is exactly the goal when you are trying to achieve a healthier and more efficient brain. If you are able to pull yourself out of the sympathetic mode, you can respond to situations with maturity and rationalism.

ESSENTIAL

Adaptogens are a twenty-first century savior. It's unlikely that the pace of life and fierce competition in the global market will subside. If you want to be on top of your game, and remain one of the modern-day warriors capable of withstanding stress, adaptogens should be in your toolkit.

Why Adaptogens?

Compared to other types of nootropics or dietary supplements, adaptogens are unique in the fact that they do not promote one particular goal. For example, if you're taking a supplement to help with sleep, you should expect it to help you sleep. That supplement could primarily only be used and recommended for times when sleep is impaired and you need a circadian rhythm reset.

Adaptogen use can address such issues as:

- Headaches
- Depression and mood disorders
- Autoimmune diseases
- Neuroprotection
- Mental stress and physical stress
- Sleep disorders and insomnia
- General immunity

All of these beneficial effects meet the requirements of the term adaptogen. They are nontoxic to the user, and normalize and benefit the entire system of the body, not just a specific ailment. Herein lies the beauty and wisdom that this group of compounds possesses.

Cholinergics

Now that you are familiar with the neurotransmitter acetylcholine, you will more easily understand the workings of a cholinergic compound. This term is frequently used in the world of nootropics to refer to a substance that interacts with the acetylcholine system.

Cholinergic substances interact with acetylcholine in different ways. For example, some may inhibit an enzyme called acetylcholinesterase. This enzyme is responsible for breaking down acetylcholine. However, sometimes too much acetylcholine is broken down and leads to reduced cognition. By taking a supplement that inhibits acetylcholinesterase, you are allowing the acetylcholine that is present to do its work, allowing you greater memory, attention, and more!

Other types of cholinergic supplements increase the sensitivity of receptors in the brain, allowing for a greater impact. The most accurate representation of cholinergics is supplements that are acetylcholine precursors. These provide the building blocks of your acetylcholine and allow a naturally higher amount of this neurotransmitter. Supplementing with precursors is the most effective and safe way to increase brain function because you're just giving the brain and body the materials it needs to create the neurotransmitters. Supplements that try to actually replicate, mimic, or replace the neurotransmitter directly can cause a down-regulatory effect, similar to how the body reduces testosterone output after taking testosterone replacement therapy.

ESSENTIAL

The mind and body know what they are doing. It's just up to you to give them some extra fuel and the right environment to thrive. If you combine some of the stress management strategies such as going for walks in nature, eating an organic, nutrient-dense diet, and then adding targeted nutrients on top of that, you'll have a recipe for success.

Cholinergic Popularity

Many companies that design and manufacture brain supplements will use substances with cholinergic properties. When you modify the acetylcholine system in any way, you are working on the systems that deal with learning, memory, and even decision-making.

By boosting the acetylcholine system in a variety of ways, you may experience:

- An increase in memory recall
- The ability to jump from one task to another without fatigue or confusion
- A lack of doubt or hesitation in decision-making
- Increased confidence and dedication to a task at hand

Researchers focus heavily on the acetylcholine system when dealing with patients suffering from Alzheimer's disease. Supplementary measures to support the natural production and protection of remaining acetylcholine in the brain are a highly recommended and necessary step to slow further degradation.

There is a difference between "regular cholinergic" and "nootropic cholinergics." For example, the compound choline found in eggs can be healthful to the brain, but it usually doesn't cause nootropic effects. Alpha-GPC is another type of choline compound that is able to penetrate the blood-brain barrier, which provides a more direct effect on the brain for enhancing brain function.

Color Enhancement

Some interesting perceptual effects of taking nootropics that act on these receptors include enhancement in colors. When taking substances that alter acetylcholine or GABA especially, colors become more vivid to the user.

While color enhancement isn't a common selling point for supplement companies, it is a relatively profound effect that can leave you in awe. Concerts, art shows, botanical gardens, or other places of natural beauty are good places to go to look for the effects of nootropics. If you are taking supplements in a sterile and boring environment, such as an office cubicle under artificial lighting, you may not have the same type of experience, even if you are taking the same compound. Pay attention to what circumstance and location you're in when taking nootropics, as it will create variation in your experience and perceived benefits.

Serotoninergics

Serotonin is what regulates mood, social behavior, appetite, and other functions such as digestion. Supplements that work on the serotonin system are called serotoninergics, and can produce effects that allow a greater sense of peace and relaxation. While the goal of serotoninergics isn't primarily to relax the user, increasing serotonin just happens to have that effect.

Serotonin deals a lot with your perception of life and events. When you balance your serotonin levels you may experience:

- An ease in learning new things
- Increased relaxation and ability to handle life
- A sense that "everything is okay"
- A reduction in anxiety, which allows more pleasure

In summary, you may feel that life itself has taken a big deep breath. You may be able to enjoy things that were previously numb to you. Your anxiety about your day-to-day tasks or the future may be lifted, allowing you to focus on the present moment. Your learning memory may feel improved, allowing you to digest research material or other fun facts that you read on the cover of a newspaper.

A popular supplement that is taken to boost serotonin levels in the alternative health community is L-Tryptophan, an amino acid that is found in turkey. And no, the turkey you eat at Thanksgiving does not calm you down and make you feel good because of the tryptophan; that theory has been disproven. Dietary consumption of tryptophan does not result in an increase in brain levels of it. More accurately, spending quality time with friends and family can calm many people down—as long as you like them, of course!

You may have some level of familiarity with serotoninergic compounds if you or someone you know has taken SSRIs since they primarily focus on altering the serotonin neurotransmitter.

Dopaminergics

You're right if you assumed that dopamine is the primary neurotransmitter when discussing dopaminergic compounds. Like acetylcholine, dopamine plays a large role in overall cognition, focus, memory, attention, and drive.

When optimized, these two neurotransmitters can make you an incredibly productive person.

When you optimize dopamine levels you may experience:

- Improved sense of clarity both visually and mentally
- Increased motivation to pursue leisure or business tasks
- Increased alertness for sports, working, and driving

In summary, you may begin cleaning up your house or reorganizing that neglected closet. You may want to work on a new project, or have a new idea, or a change in perspective on an existing idea that will allow it to become more valuable or sensible to others. Your malaise may be lifted and you may feel like you have a new lease on life.

Notice that the term "optimize" is used when discussing neurotransmitters, especially dopamine. The goal of nootropics and supplementation in general is to create balance or enhance the system to reach a healthy level. Cranking up one or more of the neurotransmitter systems can disrupt the native balance and cause anxiety or other signs of an imbalanced system.

Dopaminergic substances can be incredibly powerful for cognitive function and are commonly used for people with low libido, motivation, and drive. More serious conditions such as Parkinson's disease or other significant cognitive handicaps that relate to dopamine are where dopaminergic compounds such as L-DOPA, the precursor to dopamine, comes into play.

Anxiolytics

Anxiety is a significant issue that almost everyone has experienced at least once in life. Even if it was a short-term, situational type of anxiety, such as a speaking event or an impending financial stressor, anxiety can put a damper on how you enjoy life. Those who suffer from more chronic or unexplained sources of anxiety are at significant risk for depression, insomnia, and other degenerative effects.

Optimizing or boosting your anxiolytic response can result in a variety of effects. If we are talking about improving GABA specifically, one can experience:

- A relief from anxiety, shakiness, or other nervous tension
- Improved sleep and recovery sensation
- Less mental chatter
- Improved awareness of beauty and perception

The conventional medical treatment model for anxiety consists of prescribing a category of medication called benzodiazepines that operate on the GABA system. Low GABA levels are responsible for anxiety, nervousness, and other related symptoms. Taking a pharmaceutical substance such as Xanax can reduce the symptoms of anxiety and stress in the short term.

However, long-term use of benzodiazepines causes the body to reduce its own production of GABA, which can lead to dependence and severe withdrawal effects. People who are originally prescribed these types of medications for anxiety disorders or panic attacks may find that attempting to reduce or stop taking the drugs causes worse emotional issues than were experienced before beginning the substance.

These unsafe pharmaceutical versions of anxiolytics cause cognitive deficits and other side effects including:

- Forgetfulness
- Difficulty with coordination
- Feeling sad or empty
- Trouble concentrating
- Trouble speaking
- Trouble performing routine tasks

These are only a handful of the common side effects. The less common side effects are even more extreme and can appear as confusion about one's identity, place, and time. If the goal is optimal performance and enhanced cognitive ability, there aren't many worse substances to take.

However, the calming compounds that you will soon discover are not only useful for reducing anxiety and the tangential effects, but are completely safe and do not appear to have side effects or a risk for dependence or withdrawal effect. There could be a perceived dependence in the sense that if you feel so good taking something, why would you want to quit taking it? However, a real physical addiction characterized by the uncomfortable effects of cessation will not be something you'll have to worry about.

Finding Your Nootropic Balance

Balance is key. You are not trying to overload yourself on one particular type of compound. The goal is to determine where you are lacking most and which neurotransmitter is causing the most symptoms. Start by identifying the number of symptoms that are most burdensome to your daily life and function, and go from there.

Since you are particularly interested in cognitive enhancement and increasing your brain's power, supplementing with compounds to support dopamine, acetylcholine, and serotonin can all be helpful. GABA can't be forgotten as it creates the inhibitory balance that prevents you from too much stimulation or anxiety.

You'll learn that each day you're given in life, there may be a natural and predictable pattern for where you need more support. Genetically, you may constantly lack serotonin and feel like a dark cloud is following you every day. Your most helpful starting place may be to work on that system, since that is where the most glaring deficit is, which will allow other pieces of your life and personality to fall into place downstream.

When balance is created, increased memory, attention, learning, etc. will naturally be improved. You can specifically supplement to enhance those characteristics, but once the foundations of nutrition, lifestyle, stress management, and more are met, they will begin to improve on their own. Once you feel more human than you did before, you may be ready to experiment.

CHAPTER 5

Racetams and Synthetic Nootropics

Racetams are what generated the initial buzz that led to the explosion of interest in nootropic research and experimentation. Although humans have used natural compounds for thousands of years, there is something inherently attractive about new compounds that are created in a laboratory and vetted by scientific research. Currently, there are researchers across the globe determining what these compounds can do, why they are beneficial as nootropics, and how much any of these nootropics should be used.

Piracetam

Piracetam is the grandfather of all nootropics. It is what started the brain-boosting revolution. It works on the cellular level and has been shown to improve mitochondrial function.

What Are Mitochondria?

You probably remember learning about mitochondria in middle school biology class. Mitochondria are the powerhouse of the cell, the battery pack. Mitochondria have a powerful effect on the amount of energy in your body.

Mitochondria don't make energy out of thin air. They take nutrients from the various foods you eat and convert them into the usable form of energy known as ATP (adenosine triphosphate). This is partly why eating nutrient-poor food sabotages your energy levels. If you eat food lacking in energy, it's like trying to charge a battery when the power is out; it's not going to happen easily.

ALERT

Diseases such as chronic fatigue and fibromyalgia have to do with decreased levels of ATP, the building block of energy. The continuation of mitochondrial deficiency may end up as dementia or other forms of severe cognitive disability. The term "mighty mitochondria" is the most accurate way to remember this component of your health.

Benefits of Piracetam

If you know someone who is lacking in energy, piracetam may be the answer. It directly improves mitochondrial function and ATP production, and has been able to restore cognitive impairment in Alzheimer's patients.

Since you aren't likely to find research discussing the benefits of piracetam in healthy individuals, expected benefits include:

- Increased creativity
- Enhanced writing ability
- Improved verbal fluency

You may discover that piracetam allows you to think outside the box and helps you draw new conclusions from existing ideas. You may also discover that it becomes easier to type out your thoughts, or that the physical action of pressing fingertips on a keyboard seems smoother. Lastly, when talking in front of people for a business meeting or other social situations, words may come in rapid succession, and you may use more complex vocabulary or sentence structure than normal. You may feel more "on top of your game" in a general sense.

Pramiracetam

This smart drug is similar to piracetam and has been proven to be helpful in young males with memory and cognitive problems, specifically those suffering from head injuries in the absence of oxygen (anoxia). Other research has shown that this compound helps drug-induced amnesia, which gives promise for those recovering from anesthesia and the potentially harmful effects of pre- and post-surgery medication.

The Impact of Nitric Oxide

Research from the Medical Research Council Toxicology Unit at the University of Leicester shows that nitric oxide can improve the cognitive ability of the brain. It has been recommended for use in neurodegenerative disease. Pramiracetam has been shown to increase the level of nitric oxide in the brain, which may explain why learning and memory are improved when taking this supplement.

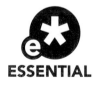

ESSENTIAL

You will discover that it's far easier to research about the older and more thoroughly studied compounds found later in this book. Some of these forms of nootropics have existed for less than a decade, so long-term study results are impossible. Remember that nootropics were designed to be safe, effective, and free from side effects. In contrast, thousands of people die each year from liver failure due to simple NSAIDs and other common over-the-counter drugs.

The research group also notes that too much nitric oxide is toxic to neurons, so a healthy balance will be necessary for the best type of treatment. This may sound like the fringe of science—and it is. For example, PubMed (*www.ncbi.nlm.nih.gov/pubmed*), a free search engine that covers life sciences and biomedical topics that is maintained by the U.S. National Library of Medicine, only shows forty-three results for the search term "pramiracetam."

Phenylpiracetam

The heavy-hitting version of piracetam is called phenylpiracetam. Notice that the only difference is the word *phenyl* in front of it. That just means that a group of atoms are added to the compound to allow it to penetrate the blood-brain barrier, making it much more effective.

The Blood-Brain Barrier

You are alive and protected from external toxins because of your blood-brain barrier (BBB). Think of it like a helmet that protects a football player from extreme head trauma. Most of the time and under the right circumstances, this barrier protects you and the player. A small hit to this barrier should be no problem. But with frequent and rough abuse of this barrier, you can experience problems.

FACT

Epilepsy is an example of what can happen when a "leaky brain" is created. Just because you have a leaky brain doesn't mean you will suffer seizures, but one of the main branches of current epilepsy research is looking at the correlation between a leaky brain and seizures.

The blood-brain barrier protects your brain from bacterial infections, various toxins, and other contaminants, and especially neurotoxic compounds that would cause damage to the central nervous system. When inflammation from diet, lifestyle, and other factors converge to cause what's known as "leaky brain," toxins that aren't supposed to pass through this protective barrier sneak through.

What does all of this leaky brain talk have to do with racetams? It's simple. When you see any supplement that begins with "phenyl," understand that this is a tactic used to increase the ability to penetrate the blood-brain barrier so that it can deliver the beneficial effects.

GABA and the BBB

For example, GABA (gamma-aminobutyric acid) supplements are readily available at most health food stores, sold to promote relaxation and to support the neurotransmitter GABA. However, this molecule is supposed to be too big to bypass the BBB. Therefore, if you take a GABA supplement and notice results from it, you may have a leaky brain. But a *phenyl*-GABA supplement will work on almost everyone because it has a free pass to head straight to the brain.

When you bypass the blood-brain barrier, you're overriding the protective mechanism designed to keep the bad guys out and let the good guys in. So make sure that what you are taking is a good and healthful product. Research all supplements carefully before taking them. Generally speaking, if it is a supplement or ingredient that mainstream companies manufacture, you can assume that it has some level of safety and benefit, but be sure to check the company's practices and history.

Phenylpiracetam and the Brain

This compound has also been shown to help those who are recovering from a stroke. Depending on the severity, strokes can lead to permanent disfigurement and disability, and successful treatment protocols are nearly non-existent in the brain department. A supplement such as phenylpiracetam may become a staple in the brain injury field in the future.

Phenylpiracetam can be a safe and potent "starter smart drug" for someone with interest in a simple but effective cognitive enhancer. It may be more expensive than piracetam, but its effects are more powerful and it requires less dosage to give the desired effect.

Other discovered benefits of phenylpiracetam are improvement of:

- Motor coordination
- Higher brain functions
- Memory
- Attention
- Counting ability

Phenylpiracetam is unique in the fact that it could fit the mold of the racetam family, but could also be considered for classification in the anxiolytic group of compounds that aid in reducing anxiety. It was found to be an effective treatment for not only depression, but also anxiety.

ALERT

Phenylpiracetam has unique properties for improving your resilience to extreme temperatures and other types of biological stressors. This substance flew under the radar for some time but was recently banned by the World Anti-Doping Agency (established in 1999 by the International Olympic Committee) due to the increased resistance to cold that this compound provides!

If you are faced with the choice of taking a compound that has few to non-existent side effects and has at least some clinical evidence for its ability to reduce depression while enhancing memory and attention, it may be something to consider before taking more dangerous alternatives. When you compare the cost of an over-the-counter compound to the costs and risks associated with more typical approaches to cognitive and mood impairments, it makes you wonder why anyone would question which route to take.

Marketing (or the lack of marketing, in the case of nootropics) is a big reason why it's a generally unknown healing modality. You may have been wondering how these compounds could be so powerful, so effective, have little to no side effects, and not be on every store shelf in the world. Within a decade or so, it could be that phenylpiracetam is a household word that is as common as aspirin.

Oxiracetam

Like all racetams, oxiracetam is not found in food or nature. It is comparable to piracetam, but is more effective for memory. It has been shown to increase cognition by 1 point on a 5-point scale with no side effects whatsoever. It has been shown to significantly reduce the symptoms of dementia and is a potent but underutilized brain-booster.

The issue with smart drugs in general is that the demographic that uses these compounds is so precise. Silicon Valley created the initial boom and interest in these compounds, primarily with young men. Research into these compounds isn't likely to be done on these groups, which decreases the published material available for you to consume.

The research that does exist is primarily focused on those who already have minor to severe cognitive deficits. One must wonder how extensive the benefits for the brain may be if the subjects used in clinical research were healthy and happy. Instead, it's just about getting back the brainpower that was lost due to aging, inflammation, damage, and other neurotoxic factors. More research is needed to determine and report the effects of oxiracetam.

Aniracetam

Aniracetam has been shown to alleviate damage done to memory and learning impairment due to trauma. It is recommended for patients who are senile or suffering other manifestations of cognitive impairment, since the current treatment model of prescription drugs ridden with side effects is lacking.

ALERT

Aniracetam is a fat-soluble compound that has a poor absorption rate of 8.6–11.4 percent. This means that if you take a dose of 100 mg, you may only absorb and utilize a tenth of that amount. This is why some companies recommend you take their product on an empty stomach to reduce the competition for absorption into the bloodstream.

In Europe, aniracetam is a prescription drug. In the United States, it is available and sold as a dietary supplement that can be found on various websites. A common brand name of aniracetam used clinically is called Memodrin. This is a true cognitive powerhouse and is highly tolerated with no side effects (except accomplishing more work in less time). It can also be used as an anti-depressant.

Other Synthetic Nootropics

The racetams are the heavy hitters of the smart drug world that most people immediately run to purchase. However, there are equally beneficial nootropics on the market that can improve your cognitive performance and generally have the same merit of being highly tolerated with no side effects.

Noopept

Noopept sounds pretty close to nootropic, doesn't it? This supplemental powerhouse is similar to piracetam, but is not considered to be in the racetam family. It is a ridiculously potent nootropic that is documented to be 1,000 times stronger than piracetam. The dosage that is generally recommended in powder form is no larger than what will fit on the head of a toothpick. You can see why education is the first step to application here!

There is clinical evidence that Noopept can reduce anxiety and the adverse effects to the brain and heart that are caused by anti-tuberculosis drugs. About one-third of the world's population has latent (or inactive) tuberculosis, meaning that they've been infected but are not (yet) ill with the disease and are not contagious. Although tuberculosis isn't common in the United States, the World Health Organization notes that in 2013, 9 million people fell ill with TB and 1.5 million of them died from the disease. Noopept may serve as not only a cognitive enhancer, but a potential lifesaver as well.

Modafinil

Modafinil has been given the most hype among the media and is likely the most prescribed smart drug on the market. It requires a doctor's authorization and is taken by adults who experience excessive sleepiness due to sleep disorders. It is commonly known as Provigil and has been commonly used for off-label use by "biohackers" to improve brain function and keep people "in the zone."

There are various and serious side effects than can occur when taking modafinil, such as a serious rash and/or allergic reaction. Some of the other side effects include depression, anxiety, headache, nausea, trouble sleeping, and back pain.

For the most part, you should steer clear of this supplement. The only reason that it is listed in this book is for educational purposes and to shine a light on a harmful substance that should be avoided whenever possible. There are far better and safer solutions to enhance your ability to focus and maintain adequate energy levels.

In clinical trials, modafinil was tolerated, but did not demonstrate any benefit for improving ADHD symptoms. It was prohibited by the World Anti-Doping Agency after several athletes were found to be using this drug to enhance performance.

In addition, this drug is considered by the military as a substitute for amphetamine, since amphetamine was typically used and best suited for times when sleep-deprived individuals were expected to have high performance.

Adrafinil

This compound is similar to modafinil, as it is also taken for its off-label supposed benefits of enhancing brain function, attention span, and more. However, it decreases your ability to sleep, and has been shown to induce orofacial dyskinesia that may persist after cessation of use. Orofacial dyskinesia is a term used for involuntary repetitive movements of the mouth and face.

ALERT

Regardless of what future studies say, adrafinil is another supplement that is only mentioned here for educational purposes and is not recommended for use. Why choose something that has risks when there are dozens of other substances that have much better track records? It's a no-brainer.

Centrophenoxine

The pharmaceutical drug called Lucidril is also known as centrophenoxine. This drug is used to treat Alzheimer's disease and help with symptoms of senility. A double-blind study of its effects on the elderly showed increased mental alertness and improved transfer of new information into the long-term memory bank.

The lead researcher at *www.Examine.com*, a site dedicated to researching and translating clinical evidence for nutrients and other compounds, had some interesting comments. The researcher, who has a BS in applied human dietetics, suggests that centrophenoxine would not need to be taken every day for life and it can yield benefits beyond simply the time it is ingested.

It can be taken as a one-time brain booster to bring the levels of attention back to normal. An interesting research document found that it reduces so-called "waste material buildup" in the brain.

L-Tyrosine

While tyrosine is lumped into the synthetic nootropic category, it is naturally found in many food sources such as fish, chicken, and pork. Tyrosine is one of many amino acids that acts as a building block of protein molecules. The body can manufacture this amino acid to support muscle tissue from another amino acid called phenylalanine.

Without enough tyrosine in the system, your thyroid can become underactive. In fact, if you're taking thyroid medication, it may not be wise to take tyrosine due to the possible interactions. Thyroid hormones are made from the combination of tyrosine and iodide. Have you heard the terms T3 and T4? Maybe you have seen them on your lab work. These are thyroid hormones that affect almost every physiological process in the body, including proper growth and development, metabolism, and heart rate.

These important thyroid hormones are a combination of tyrosine and iodide, which is why your table salt is "iodized." Long before science understood why people living away from coastal regions suffered cognitive and physical impairments, people in the Midwest and other regions suffered from goiter, a swelling of the neck that results from iodine deficiency in 90 percent of the cases. That may seem like random information, but understanding the importance of simple molecules can help millions across the world who suffer from hypo- or hyperthyroid conditions, which have become epidemic. The resulting slow metabolisms and other side effects contribute to obesity.

Tyrosine in supplemental form can be used to support the thyroid, which can aid in increasing energy and metabolism. You are basically turning up the RPM on a car when you support the thyroid. If you do this gently, you can have a nice boost of energy and may also experience the weight loss you've been searching for.

Stress and Tyrosine

Stress depletes your body and brain function on many levels, which is why some brain supplements may contain this amino acid. It has been shown to reduce the impact of acutely stressful situations such as cold temperatures and hypoxia. A trial on cadets found that during a training course, cognitive ability and blood pressure were stabilized with the help of tyrosine.

In excess, like many substances, you may experience anxiety or the feeling that you're just a bit too revved up. You may have so much energy and stimulation that you just take off and sprint down the street.

Acetyl L-Carnitine

Carnitine is a combination of amino acids that are produced by your liver and kidneys. It is naturally found in red meat, poultry, fish, and avocado, among many other protein sources. It helps the body turn fat into energy and is typically recommended as a dietary supplement for weight loss, fat burning, and physical performance. It could also be considered an anti-diabetic nutrient since it improves insulin sensitivity, and is even more helpful for cognition and performance.

Food May Not Provide the Nutrients You Need

The world of dietary supplements wants to convince people that if they just take their magic pill, potion, or powder, they don't have to eat anything. They can get all of the nutrients, protein, and other sources of nutrition from these substances. In part, they are right. The nutrient density of conventionally raised animals and produce are generally poor, and if you are taking a verified organic, grass-fed whey protein for example, you're almost better off. Of course, you aren't enjoying the chewing process like you would with a steak, but the quality of what you are taking in is improved.

You may ask, "Then why don't I just eat the foods that contain carnitine?" You should. But a portion of the population does not have adequate levels of stomach acid due to high stress, meaning their system will only partially break down proteins, fats, and other foods. Cleaving the molecules apart for absorption is a strenuous job and requires engagement of the parasympathetic mode that most people do not have. Indigestion, bloating, and other ill feelings after eating a meal can be a sign that your stomach acid levels are too low and you may need some additional support in the form of hydrochloric acid supplements.

However, for supplementing the actual nutrient you need for this application in an easily digestible form, acetyl L-carnitine can be a great way to boost your performance. It's much more readily available to the body than waiting for the steak you had at dinner to translate into mental and physical improvement.

A study in the *American Journal of Physiology - Endocrinology and Metabolism* documents the incredible capability of L-carnitine in recovering from exercise stress. Taking 2 grams of carnitine a day for three weeks resulted in greater recovery from a high-repetition squat exercise.

The brain-boosting benefits are equally impressive. A double-blind placebo study found that the particular form discussed here, acetyl L-carnitine, taken for 90 days showed significant improvement in patients with hepatic encephalopathy, which is the occurrence of confusion and altered level of consciousness caused by liver failure. You may think, "Well, I don't have liver failure, does this apply to me?" That is a hard question to answer since most studies aren't done on normal, healthy individuals. But one could assume that if sick people are helped by a supplement, healthy people should experience benefits, too.

Preventing Nootropic Side Effects

Like any supplement, drug, or even food ingredient such as gluten, there is always the potential for experiencing unwanted effects. While each person has a unique biochemistry that will result in various effects when taking a nootropic, some nutritional laws are universal.

Starting with the lowest effective dose possible is a good measure to ensure that you are maximizing your results and reducing the potential for side effects.

While side effects aren't common, they are a possibility when your body doesn't respond well to a compound or if you've simply taken too much. Since dosages depend on the compound you are using, always refer to the bottle or packaging that your supplement came with, assuming that you bought it from a reputable place that has this information listed.

If you find a compound that works for you and decide to stack one or a few more nutrients on top of it, pay close attention to the results. You may find that you are overstimulated, having passed the effective dose range and moved into territory where you can't focus at all. If you turn up the knob on a stereo system too far, for example, you will eventually blow the speakers. Use common sense and enjoy yourself as you begin to explore your options.

CHAPTER 6

Simple but Effective Nootropics

You may be feeling a bit overwhelmed—like you have just stepped into a chemistry class where the teacher fires new information your way and assumes you can digest it. Hopefully there has been an equal amount of both applicable and educational information thus far. It's time to back up just a bit and discuss some commonly known nutrients that have nootropic benefits you may have never imagined. In fact, you may have some of these in your medicine cabinet right this second.

The Importance of Minerals

Although they only make up about 4 percent of the body, minerals are some of the most important elements you need to function well. Minerals are provided solely by your food sources, which is why a proper diet rich in minerals is so important. Out of the thousands of known minerals, at least 18 of them are necessary for good health.

Minerals act as cofactors (catalysts) for enzyme reactions to keep the system functioning properly. They maintain the pH balance in your body and facilitate the transfer of nutrients across cell membranes. They play a key role in muscle health and integrity and are what allow the contraction and relaxation of muscles.

FACT

The best sources of minerals include nutrient-dense foods such as dark leafy green vegetables, mineral-rich bone broths, Himalayan salt, and mineral-rich waters. Balance is important, but generally, you need more minerals than you currently have in your system. Epsom salt baths help, too.

Dietary and Supplemental Synergy

An intelligent and healthful strategy for ensuring you have enough minerals is to combine a mineral-rich diet with smart supplementation. Unless you live on an organic farm or have direct access to nutrient-dense food within days of it leaving the soil, you will benefit from a mineral supplement. In all honesty, even those people just mentioned would benefit from mineral supplementation, because they are likely under a level of stress that depletes their minerals and vitamins anyway.

Just because a mineral is good for you doesn't mean you need to overdo it. While magnesium is an important mineral, in excess it can throw off the delicate balance of calcium and magnesium that exists. Using a methodical and gradual increase in magnesium levels is the best choice.

Magnesium

Magnesium is a cofactor, or enzyme catalyst, in more than 300 systems that regulate biochemical reactions in the body. From controlling the growth of muscle tissue to regulating your energy levels, magnesium has a hand in nearly every reaction that goes on in the body. Magnesium is also required for the synthesis of DNA, RNA, and the "master antioxidant," glutathione.

A depletion of glutathione levels is one of the most dangerous things you can endure, since glutathione is such a powerful antioxidant. In fact, low glutathione levels are observed in cancer, HIV/AIDS, trauma, burns, and athletic overtraining. Therefore, adequate levels of magnesium to support glutathione production are essential for a healthy life.

Some of the richest food sources for obtaining magnesium are almonds, spinach, cashews, and avocado. These foods should be a staple for those who want to have both a healthy brain and healthy level of magnesium. These two goals are not separate, but they depend on each other.

Magnesium Deficiency

One of the reasons that civilizations exist is because of dirt. Soil, black gold, dirt—whatever you want to call it, is the source of life. It's the root of your existence and supports your feet, farms, and cities. You can't grow food in concrete.

In fact, civilizations have crashed and burned throughout the ages due to soil and mineral depletion. If you don't allow the soil you grow food in to rest, it does not have a chance to replenish its vitamins, minerals, and other nutrients. Just because something looks like an apple doesn't mean it has the nutritional content of an apple that you need to thrive.

The solution of "no-till agriculture" has been promoted to farmers since it uses a special drill to insert seeds into the soil. This method is used in less than a quarter of cultivated areas in the United States, but is said to create a balance of soil depletion to its renewal rate.

Professor Mary Scholes and Robert Scholes have published a paper in *Science* titled "Dust Unto Dust," where they document the importance of soil quality and the survival of a civilization:

"Great civilizations have fallen because they failed to prevent the degradation of the soils on which they were founded. The modern world could suffer the same fate at a global scale. The inherent productivity of many lands has been dramatically reduced as a result of soil erosion, accumulation of salinity (salt), and nutrient depletion. [. . .] We have forgotten the lesson of the Dust Bowl: Even in advanced economies, human well-being depends on looking after the soil. An intact, self-restoring soil ecosystem is essential, especially in times of climate stress."

What does the soil have to do with magnesium deficiencies?
You can't get magnesium from your food if the soil that it is grown in doesn't have any in the first place. You can't create minerals out of thin air, so you must have a solid foundation to build on—or in this case, build in. Healthy soil creates healthy humans and vice versa.

This gives another reason to support and purchase only organic and biodynamically raised animals and produce. The organic sources have exponentially more minerals, vitamins, and other nutrients necessary for brain function in them. Early symptoms of magnesium deficiency include:

- Loss of appetite
- Fatigue
- Weakness
- Nausea
- Headaches
- Irritability
- Food cravings (especially sugar and caffeine)
- Constipation

Further and more extreme deficiencies of magnesium can manifest as anxiety and panic attacks, migraines, depression, and a failure to thrive.

Approximately 45 million Americans suffer from chronic headaches, and 28 million of them suffer from migraines. Magnesium supplementation is one of the most powerful remedies for significantly reducing migraine symptoms in clinical trails. Think before you run to the medicine cabinet; you may need to go to your supplement box instead.

A primary symptom of taking too much magnesium is diarrhea. Since magnesium generally draws water to wherever it is located, taking a large dose of it into the digestive tract can create too much water and loose stool. Just something to keep in mind before you take a large dose as you head out to a dance party!

Magnesium and the Brain

You could assume that the brain-fog epidemic is correlated with widespread vitamin and mineral deficiencies. While there are different kinds of magnesium that are better absorbed than others, it is safe to say that you need more of it.

In a study by the International Society for the Development of Research on Magnesium, it was found that there is a direct correlation between magnesium levels and cognitive function. They note that magnesium deficiency is present in several chronic, age-related diseases, including cardiovascular, metabolic, and neurodegenerative diseases.

This same group published another study to investigate the association between low serum magnesium levels and cognitive impairment in hypertensive hospitalized patients. They discovered a "significant association between magnesium imbalance and cognitive impairment," suggesting an even greater need for measuring and optimizing magnesium levels.

Forms of Magnesium

Most of the magnesium and mineral supplements you'll find at the grocery store are poorly absorbed. Magnesium oxide is a commonly supplied version because it is cheap to produce, allowing much greater profit margins for supplement manufacturers. Forms such as magnesium citrate are better absorbed, but cost more.

There are many forms of magnesium. Some are much better than others. Here is a basic overview of some of the common forms and their traits.

Magnesium Oxide

This is the most common and cheapest form of magnesium. You'll likely find this at your grocery store when searching for mineral supplements. It is poorly absorbed and of low quality overall. Take this form as a last resort, if at all.

Magnesium Citrate

This is an increasingly popular form of magnesium that is better absorbed than magnesium oxide. It has a laxative effect in higher doses, and is recommended for calming the nervous system and promoting restful sleep and general relaxation.

Magnesium Glycinate

This is a more expensive but far superior version of magnesium that does not have a laxative effect. Therefore, you can supplement with a higher dose to replenish your depleted levels without worrying about loose stools. It is a great supplement for promoting relaxation and detoxification.

Magnesium-L-Threonate

This is a new form of magnesium that is absorbed incredibly well. It is the superstar for magnesium research and benefits to the brain. While clinical human studies are limited, this new form of magnesium on the market has become a popular "nootropic mineral."

This form of magnesium is the only form that crosses the blood-brain barrier and is therefore effective for increasing the brain's magnesium levels. By increasing the brain's level of magnesium, neuro-protection and other cognitive benefits can result.

It can be helpful for reducing migraines, muscle tension, irritability, anxiety, food cravings, and sleep issues, since it is absorbed in such an efficient manner. This is a must-have supplement for your health and cognitive function.

How to Restore Magnesium Levels

There are many ways to restore magnesium, including oral and transdermal absorption. If you don't like to take pills in general or you are trying to help someone who is younger or unable to take pills, transdermal absorption is best.

You can choose to take Epsom salt baths, or engage in the more relaxing and therapeutic form of absorbing magnesium through your skin—float tanks. Also known as sensory deprivation tanks, these are essentially giant bathtubs of warm water that are loaded with an average of 1,000 pounds of Epsom salt, known as magnesium sulfate. There is about ten inches of water in the tank, enough room for you to lie down and float on the surface of the water, making you weightless. The lack of gravity from the buoyancy of the salt water allows you to float and your nervous system to relax. The side benefit is that you are absorbing magnesium through your skin, which allows your body to absorb what it needs and direct it to where it needs it most.

Pregnant women, athletes, artists, entrepreneurs, and nearly anyone and everyone who wants to relax, replenish, their mineral content and have the potential for mind expansion will benefit from these baths.

This act in itself can be considered mind-enhancing because removing the stimuli of gravity and visual input allows the brain to think freely, improving creativity, relaxation, and production of natural painkilling endorphins. Search online for a float tank center near you. They are commonly marketed as a therapy similar to a spa treatment.

Vitamin B$_{12}$

Vitamin B$_{12}$ is a crucial nutrient for your nerve health and for the production of red blood cells that carry oxygen throughout your body. Older people with vitamin B$_{12}$ levels that are lower than average are more than six times more likely to experience brain shrinkage. This brain shrinkage does not only cause cognitive deficits, but has been strongly linked with a higher risk of developing dementia at a later stage.

Vitamin B$_{12}$ deficiency is another epidemic; up to 86.5 percent of adults and elderly are deficient. Vegans are especially prone to vitamin B$_{12}$ deficiencies and even those who eat meat may be unable to properly absorb the vitamin B$_{12}$ into their system. There are many reasons for these deficiencies, but some of the most common are:

- Low stomach acid
- Acid-blocking drugs
- Excess alcohol consumption
- Nicotine

Stress could be added to the list and it would probably be correct, since it causes so many widespread effects. Vitamin B$_{12}$ deficiency doesn't just affect your energy levels, but your mood as well. For example, vitamin B$_{12}$ deficiencies are very common in those suffering mania or bipolar disorder.

An estimated 40 percent of people aged 26–83 are vitamin B_{12} deficient. It doesn't happen overnight; rather, a continual depletion of the levels is exacerbated by the biochemical effects of aging, mainly the decrease in stomach acid levels.

If you are consuming the highest-quality grass-fed beef that contains B_{12}, but are also taking a prescription acid-blocking drug, not only are you going to suffer from digestive distress, but you're likely to experience poor energy and moods as well. Optimizing your digestion is a crucial step in overall health. However, a quick and effective method of improving one's digestion is to squeeze an organic lemon into a cup with roughly 4 ounces of spring water, and drink it. The lemon juice aids in the digestive process to stimulate the existing stomach acid and break down food into usable nutrients. Digestive enzymes and hydrochloric acid supplementation can be helpful for those who are older or have a history of using proton pump inhibitors.

Eating quality sources of organic meats, and even wild game and organ meats, is a great way to optimize your vitamin B_{12} levels.

Popular Forms of Vitamin B_{12}

Like magnesium, there are some forms of vitamin B_{12} that are better than others. The following sections break down which forms of B_{12} you should seek out and which you should avoid.

Cyanocobalamin

Most commonly, you will see the cheapest and lowest quality form of vitamin B_{12} in most supplements. This is the form called cyanocobalamin. The body can't directly absorb this vitamin form; it has to convert and activate it to be usable to the body. Cyanocobalamin is a synthetic chemical that is added to supplements just to say that they have vitamin B_{12} in it.

When this cyanocobalamin is converted into the usable forms of B_{12} by the body, however, it leaves behind a cyanide ion in the body. Even though it's a minimal amount, it's best to stay away from cyanocobalamin at all costs. There are far more effective and safe supplements available.

Methylcobalamin

Methylcobalamin is one of the various "activated" forms of vitamin B_{12} that is ready for your body to put into immediate use. It is absorbed more efficiently and contains no cyanide molecule. It is commonly recommended for chronic fatigue, but offers a dual benefit of helping neurological aging, and can be especially helpful for those with extreme cognitive deficits, as in the case of Alzheimer's disease.

Since it so well absorbed, users may feel the effects rather quickly. It's best to take vitamin B_{12} in a sublingual form, to remove the chance of it not properly digesting and being absorbed into the body. The sublingual lozenge application can be a tasty treat for children or those who prefer to consume their vitamins in this manner.

Vitamin D

Vitamin D is not just a vitamin; it is a hormone that is responsible for controlling thousands of genes and processes. Vitamin D comes from a few different sources, including exposure of skin to sunlight, foods such as oily fish, and dietary supplements.

As your skin ages, it becomes less efficient at converting sunlight into vitamin D. This is when vitamin D supplementation becomes paramount. Those who live far from the equator are more likely to suffer from vitamin D deficiencies and the resulting effects.

Remember how important magnesium is? It is a vital nutrient when taking vitamin D, as it converts vitamin D into its active form. Simply taking one nutrient or the other is cutting your brain-boosting potential short. Magnesium is essential for the utilization of vitamin D, as it activates the enzymes.

ALERT

Dr. David Llewellyn at the University of Exeter Medical School found that people who were severely vitamin D deficient were more than twice as likely to develop dementia and Alzheimer's disease. Those who were severely deficient had an increase in risk to 125 percent.

Vitamin D doesn't just mean that you have a nice tan; it means that your brain is healthier, too. In fact, in *Neurology*, the official journal of the American Academy of Neurology, it was found that vitamin D deficiency is associated with a substantially increased risk of all-cause dementia and

Alzheimer's disease. Give yourself a few minutes out in the sun to absorb vitamin D before putting on a chemical-free sunscreen or covering up from the sun. Use a zinc-oxide based sunscreen for your safety.

Vitamin D Wasn't Always Low

Even after the agricultural revolution, adequate vitamin D wouldn't have been a concern for many people, as most men and women were farmers. They were outside plowing the fields and tending to their livestock.

Air conditioning wasn't around during most of the twentieth century and your grandparents likely spent their summer days on the front porch swing. They would have been exposed to plenty of natural, bright light to regulate their moods and hormones, and would have likely had adequate sun exposure to optimize their vitamin D levels.

Granted, the Inuit and those who live near the poles of the earth would never have obtained enough vitamin D from the sun, since there are months of the year where the sun may not even rise in their region. However, what these indigenous people lacked in sun exposure they made up for in their consumption of animal protein and fatty fish, providing the key nutrients and vitamins to nourish their brains.

Now it's common to hide from the sun by covering up both skin and eyes using shirts and sunglasses. The eyes are shielded from excess UV rays, which can be harmful, but they are also being kept from the biochemical reactions that give you energy, a healthy metabolism, and a bright mood.

Vitamin D and the Brain

If you have the choice to spend your free time outdoors, do it. It's better for your health and your brain. Scientists are even suggesting that mid-life crises may not be due to age, but rather the continual depletion of vitamin D levels that occur by age 40. Since the skin isn't as efficient at converting sunlight into usable vitamin D at that age, deficiencies are widespread.

Higher vitamin D levels are associated with better non-verbal, long-term memory in multiple sclerosis patients, and for this reason vitamin D has been deemed a worthwhile supplement for patients dealing with MS.

Low vitamin D levels have been linked with depression, anxiety, panic, and phobia, and supplementation should be considered when facing any medical diagnosis of these conditions.

Forms of Vitamin D

Vitamin D supplementation is rightfully becoming a staple for health seekers. Although vitamin D_3 is found nearly everywhere, there are still dozens of companies using the ineffective and low-quality vitamin D_2.

There are five forms of vitamin D, but the point of focus for the context of supplementation and optimizing your levels is the form known as vitamin D_3, or cholecalciferol. This form is inactive, but it is converted to the active form by the liver and kidneys. Most vitamin D supplements are this form, which is generally dosed at around 1,000 mg.

Take Enough but Not Too Much

The caveat for vitamin D is that you must take enough of it to actually raise your vitamin D levels. The Recommended Dietary Allowance guidelines and mainstream medical community do not recommend supplementation with vitamin D at levels that are worthy of paying attention to. Their current 400 IU recommendation is not enough to significantly raise the levels of vitamin D in the body.

Instead, you'll want to look for a 1,000 IU or even 5,000 IU dose to take daily. It's best to take these supplements in combination with vitamin K_2 and magnesium. Vitamin K_2 acts as a director for the body's calcium and prevents it from being shunted into the wrong places. You don't want calcium build up in your arteries, and vitamin K_2 and magnesium will help prevent that from happening.

Vitamin D levels can be checked by your regular doctor. You'll want your levels to be at least 50 ng/dl. It has been said that levels of 70–100 ng/dl are even better, and may result in many healthful effects such as a reduction or elimination of lower back pain, since research has correlated chronic lower back pain to vitamin D deficiency.

You'll likely notice an improvement in your mood after optimizing your levels. It's a gentle but effective supplement for your brain function. To be accurate in your supplementation, it's best to retest your levels every six months after beginning a supplement protocol to determine two things: whether your supplement is actually working, and how well it is working. Once you "max out," you can take a few months off from supplementing, then retest.

Omega-3s

Americans love their fried foods. From fried chicken to the fried Oreos you may find at the local state fair, fried foods are everywhere. The fats used in cooking and frying are typically canola oil, rapeseed, and other refined and processed omega-6 oils. These are rancid and inflammatory to the mind and body, and result in a plethora of negative effects.

The Balance Is Gone

Your fatty acids are designed to be balanced. Specifically, the omega-6 to -3 ratio is one that has gained importance in the health field in the last decade. An optimal ratio would be about 4 to 1 for omega-6 to omega-3. However, in modern cooking oils such as canola and other types of omega-6 fats, the ratio is way off, somewhere in the ballpark of 20 to 1 for some people. This imbalance and lack of omega-3 fats causes inflammation, which affects both physical and mental performance. Brain fog and brain inflammation can cause a downward spiral of effects for your cognitive ability.

Simultaneously removing (or significantly lowering) the intake of omega-6 fats while increasing the consumption of omega-3 fats is one of the most important health strategies you can implement. Whether you take supplementary measures alone or combine a diet rich in omega-3s with your supplements, the truth is that you need healthy fats to fuel your cognitive function. Without them, it will suffer.

Fats and the Brain

The good fats that are found in krill oil, for example, have been proven to improve working memory and to activate cognitive function. Even better, it has been found that these omega-3 fats protect against neurodegeneration and cognition loss.

A higher omega-3 index was correlated with a larger brain and hippocampus in postmenopausal women. It is already known that the destruction of the hippocampus is part of the reason that memory and cognitive ability begins to fail, but if one is able to increase the size and protect it with omega-3 fatty acids, there is hope.

A study from the *American Journal of Clinical Nutrition* found that DHA supplementation improved memory and reaction time in healthy young adults. For more information, go to *http://ajcn.nutrition.org/content/97/5/1134.short*. EPA was found to enhance neurocognitive function after only 30 days of supplementation. It's hard to pick a favorite, as EPA and DHA are both beneficial, and when supplementing in the form of krill oil, they come packaged together.

FACT

DHA (docosahexaenoic acid) is essential to pre- and postnatal brain development. EPA (eicosapentaenoic acid) is more influential on behavior and mood, benefiting symptoms of ADHD, autism, dyslexia, and aggression. Accelerated cognitive decline and mild cognitive impairment correlate with lowered tissue levels of DHA/EPA. Adequate omega-3 supplementation improves these symptoms.

Where to Get Healthy Omega-3s

The same ancestors who hunted and gathered wild food would have eaten plenty of fish where available. It was a rich source of protein, fat, and the extremely important omega-3 fatty acids that are almost absent in the modern diet today. These omega-3 fats are important for nourishing the brain and providing a good fuel source for energy.

There are many types of omega-3 fatty acids, but the most common three are EPA, DHA, and ALA (α-Linolenic). The most beneficial types are EPA and DHA, which come from animal sources, mainly krill and fish oil supplements. ALA is found in plant sources such as hemp or flaxseed, but less than 5 percent of these short-chain fatty acids are successfully converted (by the body) to the more beneficial long-forms of EPA and DHA.

As concerns about ocean pollution begin to rise, some people are beginning to stray away from fish and are subsequently becoming deficient in fatty acids. Luckily, you can get nearly the same amount of omega-3 fats from eating grass-fed beef as you can from salmon. This is a great relief for those who don't have access to (or simply don't want to) eat fish.

Mercury

Mercury is converted by bacteria into methylmercury, which is a toxic compound to fish and humans. The toxicity is generally found in saltwater fish; the ocean absorbs the mercury that comes from the tons of pollution created by coal-burning energy plants. China is the world's leading polluter and user of these substances. Research has found that even in the south central United States, freshwater fish has equally dangerous levels of mercury concentration as fish found off the coast of China and that fishermen should be cautious about over-consuming their catch.

The easiest and most efficient way of boosting your omega-3 levels is to take a krill oil supplement. Krill are small crustaceans that are harvested from the ocean. They are so small that the risk of toxicity is minimal. They are commonly sourced from Antarctica, and are labeled as "Antarctic krill oil." Some companies are beginning to farm these krill for harvesting, but the quality is likely lower than that found in the wild.

CHAPTER 7

Nootropics from Nature

Over a thousand years before the word "nootropic" would be coined, ancient civilizations were using substances that improved their health and well-being. Their diet was rich in compounds that helped them protect, nourish, and stimulate higher brain function. These compounds were also used in ancient ceremonies and cultural practices to promote attention, speed, and mental accuracy.

Alpha-GPC

Choline is an essential nutrient in the B-vitamin family. It is found in egg yolks, among many other dietary sources, and must be present in your diet to ensure healthy brain function. There are supplemental forms of choline that attempt to mimic the dietary component, but are not generally well absorbed.

Alpha-GPC is an exception because it can deliver choline across the blood-brain barrier with ease. An Italian multicenter clinical trial study in the New York Academy of Sciences used alpha-GPC and took over 2,000 patients suffering from a recent stroke and found that their mental recovery was substantial after taking alpha-GPC supplementation.

Choline Overview

The majority of the population is deficient in choline and suffers decreased mental performance because of it. The National Health and Nutrition Examination Survey stated that only 2 percent of postmenopausal women consume the recommended intake for choline. Brain fog and decreased mental performance are not just something that happens because you're getting older. There is likely a dietary deficiency that can be compensated for.

Choline was not considered an essential nutrient until 1998, although it had been discovered over a hundred years before that. Choline is important for normal brain function because it increases the synthesis of the neurotransmitter acetylcholine. Getting adequate levels of choline can help with your memory and attention.

Beyond postmenopausal women, people such as athletes, frequent alcohol drinkers, and those taking nootropics in the racetam family are at risk for choline deficiency and may benefit from dietary increases and/or supplementary measures.

To boost your choline levels naturally, you should consume the following organic foods:

- Eggs (yes, eat the yolk)
- Broccoli
- Spinach
- Almonds
- Chicken

The Need for Choline

When people are taking nootropics such as piracetam, aniracetam, etc., they depend on a rich source of choline for the brain to function properly. The more powerful nootropics in the racetam family tend to deplete the levels of choline in the brain, which can cause headaches and other mildly uncomfortable symptoms related to the reduction in levels of choline and acetylcholine. Choline is the building block for acetylcholine, so if you are not obtaining the raw materials necessary to produce it, you might notice it as poor focus and concentration, slow and confused thinking, and a lack of joy.

If you take regular choline supplements, the best form to boost your choline level in your brain is alpha-GPC since it is so potent and effective. If you supplement and end up with too much choline, you may notice other mild side effects, such as jaw tension. You may find yourself rubbing your jaw to relieve a sense of fullness or achiness there. If this happens, cut down on your alpha-GPC intake.

Alpha-GPC is a safe, effective, and pleasant supplement to start with if you are overwhelmed with all of your options. It has a direct link to brain performance and has been proven to enhance cognitive performance in those who are affected by mild to moderate dementia.

Stacking, or combining alpha-GPC with any racetam, is a good way to maintain levels of acetylcholine in the brain. There is a balancing act that exists with neurotransmitters, and to stay on top of your game in the long run you will need to be sensitive to the subtle changes in your cognitive abilities that occur when tweaking any supplement protocol.

Alpha-GPC is not just a good supplement to take alone or with racetams. It can be taken in combination with nearly any supplement you find in this book. It is not considered a heavy-hitter, but rather a gentle and effective way to optimize a key system in the brain—the acetylcholine system.

Phosphatidylserine

Phosphatidylserine (PS) is a nutrient that is part of your cell membrane. It is found in neurons and nerve cells, and plays a key role in memory and overall cognition. Phosphatidylserine is a protector of these cells and carries messages between them. It's difficult to obtain adequate amounts from your food, which is why many people supplement with it.

Phosphatidylserine supplements were once typically sourced from bovine brain, but fear about mad cow disease significantly reduced the demand and caused a major shift in the way they were sourced. Scientists discovered that soy lecithin actually has over 5,000 mg of phosphatidylserine per 100 grams, compared to only 713 mg per 100 grams in bovine brain. This new source of phosphatidylserine quickly became the new gold standard for the dietary supplement market.

Concerns about consuming soy have gained popularity in the health field due to the potential for allergy and estrogenic effects. Luckily, you do not have to depend on soy lecithin for obtaining phosphatidylserine. Specialized manufacturers have recently derived the same therapeutic compound from sunflower lecithin! Look at your label source when making a purchase.

How People Had a Good Memory Before Supplements

When you see the amount of supplements that are helpful for brain function, energy, exercise performance, and more, it makes you wonder how humans were able to survive and thrive before the pill-popping era. One must remember that the original human diet was far different than today's standard American diet.

The reason that phosphatidylserine is so effective for boosting brainpower is because it contains both amino acids and fatty acids. DHA is a key component naturally found within the molecule. It can be a perfect addition and complimentary nutrient to combine with krill oil, simultaneously balancing the omega-6 to omega-3 ratio while improving brain function.

Generations that would have consumed pig and bovine brain as part of their diet are passing. Some who lived through the Great Depression understood that every part of an animal was important and should not be wasted.

This same mentality could have been borrowed from certain aboriginal beliefs that one should use every part of an animal from nose to tail, both for overall health and respect for the animal.

The nutrient density of the modern diet is lacking in so many ways, that even if one began to eat bovine brain again, it's uncertain how much nutrition it would contain and, more importantly, how it would taste. Fortunately, supplementation methods have been refined so much that a simple gel capsule is typical for taking phosphatidylserine.

What Can Phosphatidylserine Do for You?

There are several thousand studies on phosphatidylserine showing benefits in rat and human trials. Some of the most notable benefits of supplementation include, but are not limited to:

- Improved memory
- Increased concentration
- Increased attention
- Improved learning ability
- Boost in mood (primarily fights depression)
- Preventing exercise and stress damage
- Balanced cortisol

A study from *Clinical Interventions in Aging* found that supplementation with soybean-derived phosphatidylserine 300 mg a day, significantly improved memory recognition, memory recall, executive functions, and mental flexibility. A side benefit was a reduction in both systolic and diastolic blood pressure and significant improvement in total learning and immediate recall.

ALERT

Are you someone who forgets a person's name as soon as they tell it to you? "Hi, I'm . . . ." It's just gone from your brain. Phosphatidylserine significantly improves the type of memory required for these scenarios. If you are preparing to go to an important event where name recall is of the upmost importance, supplementing for 6–12 weeks ahead of time is advised.

The HPA Axis

The HPA axis, sometimes referred to as the HPTA axis, is a system that operates in a complex manner to trigger the stress response. By releasing various chemicals to respond to the stressors, your body is "switched on" and ready to go. This response happens in less than a second in some cases, leaving you sweating and white-knuckled on your steering wheel in five o'clock traffic. This response heightens your senses such as vision and hearing, and allows your muscles to fill up with blood to fight-or-flight your stressor.

The HPA axis also controls digestion, the immune system, and, for the context of this book, mood and emotions. It's important to have a basic understanding of the endocrine glands involved in your fight-or-flight response, because phosphatidylserine acts upon this system in a beneficial way.

Hypothalamus

The first letter H stands for hypothalamus, a small portion of the brain that links the nervous system with the endocrine system. It's nearly centrally located in the brain above the brain stem and is the size of an almond in humans. This tiny gland is responsible for some of your metabolic processes, such as body temperature, hunger, thirst, fatigue, sleep, and circadian rhythms. In short, it's one of the most important parts of the brain to keep your life and body operating in a normal fashion.

The hypothalamus "listens" in a way; it is responsive to stress, hormones, steroids, pheromones, and light, meaning that the seasons and sleep cycle coordinate with it. You could assume that using excess artificial light at nighttime, especially during the winter months, throws off the hypothalamus's delicate balance and circadian rhythm that keeps you operating at 100 percent efficiency.

Pituitary

The pituitary gland is an even smaller (but equally important) component of the brain. It is the size of a pea in humans and plays a role in growth, blood pressure, certain sex organs and metabolic functions, temperature regulation, and pain relief.

The front (or anterior) portion of the pituitary secretes hormones such as human growth hormone (HGH), thyroid-stimulating hormone (TSH), adrenocorticotropic hormone (ACTH), and beta-endorphin. There are other hormones, such as the "cuddling hormone" called oxytocin, which are also produced by the pituitary.

People who have an excess of growth hormone causing gigantism have an impaired or diseased pituitary gland. It's amazing to think that an alteration or dysfunction in a gland the size of a pea can create humans who are seven feet tall or more. This also suggests that attempting to modify this system by using steroids or growth hormones without a doctor can be risky and flat-out dangerous.

Adrenals

Last in the HPA axis are the adrenal glands. You have two of them, one that sits on top of each kidney. They are not in the brain, obviously, but they play arguably the most important role in the system, which is to produce even more hormones such as cortisol, DHEA, adrenaline, and dopamine.

Where It Goes Awry

The HPA axis is thrown off by many things, including stress and poor sleep. If you are able to wake up and go to bed with the sun, do it. This is good insurance for regulating this system. It isn't foolproof, of course, because a poor diet containing sugars and processed foods lacks the nutrients necessary for optimal function.

The combination of mental, emotional, physical, and nutritional stressors combine to create something commonly referred to as "adrenal fatigue." This has become a buzzword in the last few years, and people across the globe are self-diagnosing themselves with this health problem. It's actually a safe diagnosis to give yourself, because it's likely that all modern-day humans are experiencing at least mild adrenal fatigue.

HPA axis dysregulation is evident in depressed, bipolar, and anxious people. This is the result of a nervous system that has switched into an inflammatory, stressed state. The neurotransmitters are thrown out of balance, which can have many effects.

One with HPA dysregulation or adrenal fatigue may experience:

- Changes in sleep pattern
- Loss of energy
- Loss of motivation

- Changes in appetite
- Inability to handle stress
- Food cravings and binge eating
- Trouble concentrating

This list of symptoms could easily triple or quadruple, but the fact remains the same: Addressing adrenal fatigue and HPA axis dysregulation with a nutrient-dense diet and smart supplementation, including phosphatidylserine, is of the utmost importance.

Phosphatidylserine Benefits

In a supplement trial using 75 healthy male volunteers divided into low-stress and high-stress groups, it was found that the high-stressed individuals attained a normal range of cortisol with phosphatidylserine supplementation. There was not a significant change in the low-stress group, likely because their cortisol wasn't high to begin with.

Attention-deficit hyperactivity disorder (ADHD) is the most commonly diagnosed behavioral disorder of childhood. Research from the *Journal of Human Nutrition and Dietetics* investigated whether supplementation with soy-derived phosphatidylserine (PS) improved ADHD symptoms in children. It was found that short-term auditory memory, inattention, and impulsivity were all improved and no adverse side effects were observed. PS supplementation is a safe and natural nutritional strategy for improving mental performance in both adults and young children suffering from ADHD.

An equally interesting study from a medicine and exercise science journal investigated the effects of PS on markets of oxidative stress and muscle damage initiated by intermittent exercise that mimics soccer play. It was found that PS did not blunt the cortisol response, and the time it took to become exhausted increased.

Although PS wasn't able to blunt the cortisol response, research from the *International Journal of Sport Nutrition and Exercise Metabolism* found that 600 mg of PS supplementation was an effective supplement for combatting exercise-induced stress and preventing the physiological deterioration that can accompany too much exercise. PS supplementation promotes a healthy hormonal status for athletes by blunting increases in cortisol levels.

It is important to remember that studies generally look at a small group of people and in the case of these two journals, you are only hearing results from a total of 26 male subjects. Just because one study says that cortisol isn't blunted from PS supplementation and the other says the opposite doesn't mean that you shouldn't try it for yourself.

The effects of cortisol on the mind and body are the same whether you are discussing exercise-induced cortisol spikes or the stress from your boss in an office setting. Cortisol can successfully be managed with nutrients and a reframing of the stressor that you are facing. Combining both self-psychology and self-experimentation makes sense.

The reason that phosphatidylserine is so effective at protecting the nerve cells in the brain, improving cognitive function, increasing memory and recall, improving focus and attention, concentration, and the ability to communicate is that it crosses the blood-brain barrier and safely reverses any biochemical alterations and structural deterioration that impair neurotransmission.

Another helpful but hard to convey benefit of PS is that it reduces the amount of fatigue perceived by the person taking it. One person may go under the same amount of stress as someone else, but his perception of it feels less significant. Whether this effect is a physiological or biological response, it doesn't matter; having the power over your stress, even in your mind, is a powerful thing.

Creatine

Creatine is a naturally occurring chemical that supplies energy to all cells in the body. Approximately 95 percent of creatine is stored in skeletal muscle. It can be obtained from foods such as fish and meats, which is why vegetarians are likely low in creatine.

Creatine monohydrate is one of the most commonly ingested and researched sports supplements on the market and is a popular component of many athletic and bodybuilding products. It is especially helpful for weightlifters and football players, since the energy demands are so high for these groups. Higher amounts of creatine in skeletal muscle increase the amount of energy output available.

Creatine is also used for cognitive deficits such as depression, bipolar disorder, and Parkinson's disease. It is also recommended to supplement with creatine to slow the worsening of Lou Gehrig's disease, also known as ALS.

Creatine plays a pivotal role in brain energy homeostasis and has been shown in supplemental trials to significantly improve both working memory and intelligence tasks that require speed of processing.

Boosting the Effects of Creatine

Most creatine supplements will be labeled with the advice to consume with simple carbohydrates (such as juice) to provide glucose (sugar), which helps creatine uptake. This just means that drinking juice and taking a creatine supplement together can enhance the effects. However, juices can spike your insulin levels, which can result in hypoglycemia, mood swings, and type 2 diabetes in frequent, long-term, and excessive consumption.

A healthier and more rational way to get the most out of your creatine supplement is to take fenugreek with it. Fenugreek is an herb that is popular as a culinary spice among the Mediterranean community.

It has been found that taking creatine with fenugreek in the form of seed extract resulted in significantly increased absorption and performance. This herb gives the same effect as glucose, but without the harmful side effects of sugar. Fenugreek actually balances blood sugar, which can result in a mild mood-stabilizing effect as well.

Vegetarians Need Even More Creatine

Since creatine is sourced naturally from meats, vegetarians are at the most risk for creatine deficiency. In terms of improving brain function, it was found that vegetarians taking creatine supplements had improved memory and processing of information.

The obvious remedy is to eat organic and grass-fed meats, but some prefer to "fix" a vegetarian diet by taking various supplements and compounds to make up for the components lacking in the diet. Remember that a vegetarian diet may be healthful for a short amount of time to help people detox or to heal themselves from a certain health situation, but animal proteins, fish, or other types of creatures must be consumed for optimal health and longevity.

If you need more information regarding the negative impacts of a vegetarian diet, please read *Nutrition and Physical Degeneration* by Weston A. Price to learn about the hunter-gatherer tribes around the world and how not one vegetarian culture was healthy. Although the original publication of this book dates back to the late 1930s, there are timeless and inflexible dietary laws that were observed. Those who had a mixture of plants and animals without refined sugars were the healthiest people of all.

ESSENTIAL

Consider Dr. Price's book an essential read for yourself and your friends and family. Historical information about the health and diet of humans before processed foods took over will only increase in importance as time passes. Ask your grandparents about the "good ol' days of food," if you are still blessed with their presence.

L-Theanine

Theanine is an amino acid naturally found in green tea. It was found to be a constituent of green tea in 1949, which has been used for thousands of years for its benefits without knowing what was in it. It's interesting how science is good at identifying compounds, but ancient people had discovered the benefits of foods or beverages containing them long before the research existed.

You may recognize that green tea and yoga go well together. This is not a coincidence, as green tea is helpful for achieving a heightened state of awareness and improving overall cognitive function and performance. Green tea's theanine component is able to effectively cross the blood-brain barrier, giving it great effectiveness with just one cup.

Research has found that theanine content in green or black tea is typically around 20 mg, which is not enough to create alpha brain waves. Alpha brain waves are said to be the connector between the conscious and subconscious mind. Being in an "alpha state" is one where you can identify your subconscious thoughts and observe them. This is often the goal of a meditative practice. To successfully get into the alpha state, or to produce alpha brain waves to enhance your creativity and focus capabilities, you'll need more than just a cup of green or black tea.

To improve your brain function effectively by drinking tea, you will need a type of tea called matcha. As mentioned earlier, matcha tea comes from the same plant as green tea, but it is grown in a special manner to greatly increase the amount of theanine in the leaves. Matcha is shaded from the sun, which causes the plant to turn a darker color and increases theanine content, making the tea more potent in taste and effect. It has many more antioxidants than standard green tea. Preparing and consuming matcha tea is different, too, as you consume the entire leaf that is ground up and stirred into hot water, as opposed to steeping a tea bag and removing it.

Matcha tea has been part of Japanese culture for over a thousand years, but has appeared in the popular American market only recently. Commercial coffeehouse chains such as Starbucks now offer matcha drinks to their loyal customer base. However, it's best to stay away from the Starbucks standard matcha latte that packs a whopping 55 grams of sugar into a 16-ounce cup. Talk about a way to ruin the health benefits of a naturally healthful drink.

Matcha Quality

There are several grades of matcha tea that determine the effectiveness and overall quality. The highest grade would be labeled as an organic grade A ceremonial tea. This ensures that your product is free from added chemicals and pesticides, and meets the highest standards of tea quality. If you are looking to drink matcha by itself, you want that grade.

Branching off from the most expensive class of matcha you'll find organic grade B and C powder. These are still of high quality, but may lack the potent taste and bright green color that you'll find in the premium version. It still contains theanine and will noticeably improve your mood, focus, and attention, while giving you a sense of peace.

If you are unable to find a certified organic matcha tea, look for one that is considered a ceremonial grade powder. This is a high standard that would probably taste good on its own. If you compared these teas with a matcha tea product with no mention of organic or ceremonial grade on the label, you would notice the difference. The lower-quality matcha tea powders can be used in ice cream, smoothies, and other recipes that call for the addition of matcha for taste or color. Just don't expect to enjoy drinking a low-quality powder by itself.

Theanine Benefits

Theanine has been used in clinical practice for anxiety, panic, OCD, and bipolar disorders as it calms the nervous system gently but effectively. This isn't a type of compound that is going to mimic a prescription anxiety reliever such as Xanax, but it can provide a gentle relaxing effect. Since theanine is gentle in nature, it can be taken during the morning or afternoon with no fear of falling asleep on the job.

Some consider theanine as a required ingredient to mix with caffeine because it balances out the effects. Someone who drinks coffee and becomes too overstimulated will benefit from theanine supplementation. The typical ratio to mix them is 2 parts theanine to 1 part caffeine. If you take a small cup of coffee that contains 100 mg of caffeine, you'll want to take 200 mg of theanine with it to balance it out. There are no risks for theanine, so feel free to create your own ratio; this is just what's commonly recommended.

In the *Journal of Medicinal Food*, it was found that a combination of green tea extract and theanine resulted in improved memory and selective attention. The brain waves called theta waves are an indicator of cognitive alertness and were significantly increased in multiple parts of the brain. This combination is a great intervention for cognitive improvement.

Theanine blocks the binding of L-glutamic acid to glutamate receptors in the brain, which is part of the reason that it is calming and stabilizing to one's mood and nervous system. The anti-stress benefits were measured in subjects that took orally administered theanine. A side benefit aside from the calming and cognitive enhancement of theanine is a reduction in blood pressure.

Recent research has picked up on the trend of combining caffeine and theanine and found that both 10 minutes and 60 minutes after consumption of this mixture, attention was significantly improved, but not alertness. However, many of the other compounds that you may be stacking with theanine and caffeine can improve alertness.

College students and high-performing Silicon Valley employees have popularized the use of nutrients and drug compounds for cognitive performance. However, the emphasis on increasing performance and "cranking up the brain" have led some to burn out, or to go too long without eating a meal because they are so focused. Theanine would be a great nutrient to balance out this over-stressed and overworked lifestyle.

University students in school to become a pharmacist are probably some of the most stressed individuals. A small study took these students and gave them an intervention of 200 mg of theanine supplementation. This was taken after breakfast and lunch for one week prior to the practice and continued for ten days in the practice period. To be as accurate as possible, salivary amylase was sampled (as opposed to relying on perception of stress), which measures sympathetic nervous system activity. Theanine supplementation resulted in lower levels of this measurement, indicating a relaxed nervous system.

FACT

Theanine has been shown to increase the alpha band (8–14 Hz) during electroencephalographic (EEG) readings in humans. Alpha band activity is a key component of selective attention processes. Alpha wave training is used for overcoming phobias and to calm down hyperactivity during biofeedback training. Theanine has clear psychoactive properties that represent a naturally occurring compound used in the brain's attentional system.

Citocoline

Citocoline is a naturally occurring compound that is necessary for the synthesis of phosphatidylcholine, an important phospholipid for the brain. Citocoline is able to cross the blood-brain barrier and gets nearly immediate access to the bloodstream, resulting in noticeable benefits and changes in perception very quickly. Some may notice the effects of citocoline within the first couple hours of taking it.

Effects of citocoline are an enhancement in multiple neurotransmitter systems including dopamine, norepinephrine, and acetylcholine, hence the name "coline." You can expect your vision to become more acute when taking citocoline. It may seem as if you have mild "HD vision" and that colors are brighter, sharper, and more enjoyable to look at. It may be a good supplement to use when visiting an art gallery!

Citocoline Research

So far, there haven't been a lot of studies done on the effects of cito-coline. Research documents the neuroprotective action of citocoline in the brain, which is beneficial in some slowly advancing neurodegenerative disorders such as glaucoma and mild vascular cognitive impairment. A toxic diet, excess stress, and pollution all contribute to inflammation, which may contribute to cognitive impairment. It's safe to say that nearly all humans would benefit from taking citocoline.

Citocoline is made up of choline and cytidine, which are readily absorbed by the gastrointestinal tract and blood-brain barrier. This could be why its effects are noticeable so quickly. Gastrointestinal absorption is something to keep in mind when experimenting with supplements. Competition in the gut in the form of food can lead to diminished results. If you are sensitive to most supplements and drugs, it may be better for you to consume these supplements with a snack to give a slower rise in effects.

The *Clinical Interventions in Aging* held a citocoline supplement trial in 265 patients who were 65 years old or older. Citocoline was effective and tolerated well in patients with mild cognitive impairment, and it was also found that brain metabolism was increased, resulting in a more active central nervous system. In layman terms, it gets the brain and nervous system turned up and causes an increase in the production of neurotransmitters, leading to improved mood and cognition.

CHAPTER 8

Earth-Grown Nootropics

Mushrooms, flowers, and trees aren't just for looking at with awe. Some cultures have eaten mushrooms for health benefits and general enjoyment for over a thousand years, and recent research has highlighted certain species that benefit the brain more than you could have imagined. You will never look at plants and fungi the same way after you discover their safe but potent brain-boosting effects such as increased attention and even protection from radiation.

Reishi

Reishi is commonly known as *Lingzhi* in Chinese. It is an herbal mushroom that is non-toxic and can be taken daily to regulate the immune system. There are several components of mushrooms that give them medicinal value such as polysarrharides, triterpenoids, proteins, and amino acids. These different components have various effects such as treating anxiety, reducing stress, and lessening fatigue.

Reishi is an incredibly bright red mushroom that was first documented as used medicinally during the Han Dynasty in 206 BCE. Reishi roughly translates to "super mushroom," and has been shown to suppress the growth of breast cancer cells and allow for detoxification of harmful heavy metals that accumulate in the body.

Reishi is usually not eaten since it can be tough and bitter. Instead, it can be ground or extracted into a liquid tincture, which provides far more beneficial compounds without having to eat a mushroom the size of your hand. Reishi capsules are commonly found at health food stores and are expected to become more readily available as health-conscious consumers begin to discover the immense benefits.

Historically, reishi would have been prepared in the form of tea or other infusion. Some companies today sell mushroom teas, and also add reishi to coffee and chocolate bars for a true superfood mixture. Keep your eyes peeled for reishi to be the next ingredient addition at your favorite local grocery.

Reishi Effects

You should expect to notice the effects of reishi within two weeks of supplementation. It can significantly improve your well-being after a month or two of continuous supplementation. Some call reishi "the mushroom of immortality," although credible research on extending lifespan is currently nonexistent. One study from the *International Journal of Medicinal Mushrooms* did find that reishi extract significantly enhanced healing activity in wounds when applied topically in an ointment preparation. It might be time to add some to your first-aid kit in capsule and liquid extract forms for internal or external applications.

In terms of brain health and cognitive performance, research is based primarily on clinical experience. Learning and memory can be enhanced when taking reishi. It has been found to reduce neuronal cell death and to relieve cell injury. You can find a bottle of reishi capsules for less than $10 online. Inexpensive products aren't of much interest to research groups due to lack of potential profits, unlike pharmaceutical drugs. This is the beautiful thing about inexpensive compounds like reishi; you are able to feel and experience the results for yourself.

Reishi has antidepressant effects when used in extract form and also protects against liver damage. Reishi protects your memory center, the hippocampus, and helps regulate blood sugar for those who tend toward hypo or hyperglycemia. Those who are in the pre-diabetes category may benefit from reishi supplementation to reduce the possibility of becoming a full-blown diabetic. Lastly, reishi has been shown to protect against liver damage and to be an incredibly healthful tool for those who are undergoing chemotherapy and/or radiation, or are frequently exposed to airborne toxins, or consumable toxins like alcohol. One day you might even find reishi in a hangover recovery formula.

Lion's Mane

Lion's mane is a mushroom variety that looks much different than other mushrooms. If you can picture pom-poms that cheerleaders use, you understand the shape and look of lion's mane. Lion's mane in Latin is called *Hericium erinaceus*, which roughly translates to "hedgehog." Some also call lion's mane the bearded tooth mushroom.

ALERT

There were no animals harmed in the making of this compound! Lion's mane is the common name for one of the most interesting-looking fungi in existence and holds great potential as a mushroom superstar. This bright white, globular-shaped mushroom is covered in dangling spines.

One of the world's leading experts on medicinal mushrooms, Paul Stamets, says that lion's mane can taste like lobster or shrimp, and that it's best to consume it when it's caramelized in olive oil, deglazed with sake wine, and finished with butter to taste. It can be bitter if not cooked until crispy along the edges.

Typically, lion's mane will be found and consumed in capsules, and is becoming a popular mushroom for its nootropic effects. It is native to North America, Europe, and Asia, and grows in late summer and fall on trees such as the American beech. You can safely harvest it from the forest yourself as long as you know what you're looking for. It's a very distinct-looking mushroom, so chances picking a wrong one are unlikely. Realistically, however, most people don't have or want that opportunity; if you are looking to buy it, seek out wild harvested or organically grown lion's mane whenever possible.

Lion's Mane Benefits

This edible mushroom contains a class of compounds that stimulates the production of nerve growth factor (NGF). NGF is a small protein that is important for the growth, maintenance, and survival of brain cells. Lion's mane increases levels of NGF, leading scientists to believe that it can have some effects on brain function and the nervous system.

A 2010 study from a biomedical research journal in Tokyo, Japan took thirty females and gave them cookies containing either lion's mane mushrooms or a placebo. A reduction in depression and anxiety were found in the group that consumed the lion's mane cookies. For more information, go to *www.ncbi.nlm.nih.gov/pubmed/20834180*.

FACT

There are many synergies in the world that can enhance the effects of supplements. A 2015 journal entry in the *Archives of Physiology and Biochemistry* documented the neuro-protective effects of lion's mane enriched with garlic extract. It was found that neuro-protection was enhanced by 50 percent when garlic extract was consumed with the lion's mane. This combination also decreased p21 gene expression by 70 percent, a gene that is normally "activated" when tumors are present in humans.

Nerve injury can lead to numbness, pain, and other effects that are uncomfortable to live with. A 2015 study in the *Chinese Journal of Integrative*

Medicine found that an aqueous extract of lion's mane used in the treatment of nerve injury in rats was successful.

More specifically, in 2013 the *Journal of Complementary and Integrative Medicine* outlined the various medicinal benefits from the components of the lion's mane mushroom: the polysaccharides are responsible for anti-cancer, immuno-modulation, antioxidant, and neuro-protection.

Adrenal Recovery and Cognitive Performance

Adrenal fatigue is a major factor for sugar cravings, fatigue, irritability, and poor cognitive abilities in adults. If your goal is to enhance your cognitive ability, you can use a one-two punch by supporting the adrenal glands and the brain at the same time. Lion's mane possesses this ability and has been verified by research to increase cognitive performance scores.

A 2009 study by *Phytotherapy Research* held a double-blind, placebo-controlled trial, the best and most valuable type of test available in scientific research, on 50–80-year-old Japanese men and women diagnosed with mild cognitive impairment. The subjects took 250 mg tablets of lion's mane powder three times a day for 16 weeks. As early as 8 weeks into the trial, the mushroom supplementation group showed significantly increased scores on their cognitive function tests. However, after a month of stopping supplementation, the scores decreased significantly with no other adverse effects.

Unlike some other nootropics, lion's mane is one that seems to require continuous supplementation to reap benefits.

FACT

Some research would be considered unethical if it were done on humans. Many of the studies and findings that you hear about are done on rats. This is the way that science has compared and translated benefits over to humans. It might not always directly correlate or create the exact same effects when you repeat the study in humans, but it's generally an accurate representation of what should happen.

In a study using a liquid broth of lion's mane, lion's mane was found to enhance the growth of adrenal nerve cells in rats. If you try a lion's mane supplement for yourself and notice that your stress response is improved, you may be experiencing the same effect found by these scientists. Adrenal health directly correlates to the responsiveness of your brain, and "weak adrenals" can significantly impair your ability to focus on the task at hand.

Cordyceps sinensis

Cordyceps is a genus of fungi that includes about 400 species. Specifically, *Cordyceps sinensis* is a medicinal mushroom that has been used for at least 2,000 years. It was typically sourced from the wild and until recently has only been available that way, as *Cordyceps sinensis* cultivation was not achieved until 1972.

Creating a widely available mushroom product is not easy when you depend on wild-sourcing your ingredients. Isolating a specific strain of *Cordyceps sinensis* was necessary to safely and effectively provide a product that would work. The first three strains of *Cordyceps sinensis* isolated were named CS-1, CS-2, and CS-3. The problem with them is that their growth was slow and commercial cultivation would be nearly impossible. Eventually, the popular strain used today, CS-4, was chosen, which grows very fast.

Each strain of mushroom has different characteristics in their growth rate and their medicinal value. It was the CS-4 strain that made purchasing high quality *Cordyceps sinensis* mushrooms at your local grocery store possible. If you don't have local access to *Cordyceps sinensis*, you can easily find it online. Ensure that you seek out the CS-4 strain; this should be on the label or mentioned in the sales description of a product.

Cordyceps sinensis Benefits

While human studies on cognitive performance enhanced by *Cordyceps sinensis* are rare, it has been proven that it improves learning and memory in rats, which has something to do with its action on acetylcholine receptors.

Cordyceps sinensis is quickly gaining popularity in the fitness industry due to its effects on exercise performance. A 2010 study in the *Journal of Alternative and Complementary Medicine* found that the CS-4 strain supplemented for 12 weeks increased exercise performance in healthy elderly people aged 50–75.

If you're interested in cognitive performance, you'd probably like to boost your physical potential as well. Since physical activity is capable of improving cognitive function as a side effect, lumping *Cordyceps sinensis* into the nootropic category may be a fair assessment.

As time goes on, you will be able to experiment with mushroom complexes such as lion's mane and *Cordyceps sinensis* together and report the benefits on the Internet. Since the world of nootropics and increased performance via fungi is a relatively new thing to the Western world, it's up to you to be some of the first to lead the way.

Just don't go into the woods seeking mushrooms for performance and eat them. There are many poisonous ones out there that can cause ill effects or even death. Fear not, however, as these fungi specifically mentioned here have been studied and used by ancient cultures for longer than you can track your genealogy.

For athletes, hikers, mountain climbers, or those who have a physically demanding job, *Cordyceps sinensis* can be a great addition to your supplement stack. If you are able to reduce your fatigue and are able to exercise more often or more efficiently, you could say that you're enhancing your brain, too!

Vinpocetine

Vinpocetine is a health supplement that originates from the periwinkle plant. Like other highly effective brain supplements, vinpocetine is able to cross the blood-brain barrier and increase blood flow in the brain, leading to improved cognition. Vinpocetine is a complex nootropic, and the mechanism of action is not well identified. Vinpocetine is available as a supplement by itself, but many companies have decided to use vinpocetine as an ingredient to mix with other compounds for an increased effect.

A 2014 study in the *Annals of Medical and Health Sciences Research* that included patients with cognitive impairment showed that taking a 5 mg dose twice a day for 12 weeks was enough to improve memory and concentration.

Vinpocetine gives such great benefits because it acts in a few different ways. It has anti-inflammatory qualities, which can help improve the function of the mind and body. The antioxidant and vasodilating properties are likely the most potent effects that create an improvement in cognition when supplementing with this compound. Neuroimaging studies have shown an increase in cerebral blood flow, which is especially important for those who have (or know someone who has) cerebrovascular disease, which affects 200,000 to 3 million people a year in the United States.

Vinpocetine for Memory

In one study in the *European Journal of Clinical Pharmacology*, twelve healthy female volunteers received various amounts of vinpocetine and were put through a battery of psychological tests that would analyze their memory and reaction time. Among the various dosages, 40 mg was most effective at significantly improving memory. Since vinpocetine is not absorbed easily, you may need a higher dose closer to the 40 mg mark than the 5 mg dose that is commonly found.

If you want to take vinpocetine to enhance your memory, start with the minimal, 5 mg dose and take it in isolation. If you supplement with it consistently two or three times per day for a few weeks and don't notice any benefit, at that point you could probably benefit from adding in additional supplements or upping the dosage amount.

Ginkgo biloba

Ginkgo biloba supplements are among the best-selling herbal compounds in Europe and the United States. Ginkgo leaves possess chemicals known as flavonoids and terpenoids. These are antioxidants that can quench free radicals that contribute to an aging mind and body.

Unfortunately, ginkgo's very existence is at risk. When you think of threatened species, you immediately picture tigers, leopards, and other large mammals being chased out of their habitat. But plants and biological species are at great risk as well. Deforestation and climate change are a source of concern to botanists and other researchers; there are likely still thousands of undiscovered natural medicines in the Amazon rainforest and elsewhere that may never be utilized or even found.

The International Union for Conservation of Nature (IUCN) was founded in 1948 as a way to give a voice to otherwise voiceless species around the world. Their goals are to provide scientifically based information on the status of species and subspecies at a global level, to draw attention to the importance of threatened biodiversity, to influence national and international policy and decision-making, and to provide information, which guides actions to conserve biological diversity. They are an organization that you should make yourself familiar with.

The IUCN Red List of Threatened Species was founded in 1964 and is the organization's most important work. This red list discusses the most at-risk species on the planet and categorizes their conservation status ranging from lower risk to threatened, vulnerable, endangered, critically endangered, extinct in the wild, and totally extinct. The *Ginkgo biloba* tree is a living fossil that is unfortunately found on the IUCN endangered species list.

The *Ginkgo biloba* tree is called a living fossil, as recognizably similar fossils have been found dating back 270 million years. They are some of the longest-living trees on earth; some are estimated to be more than 2,500 years old. Ginkgo trees are highly prized and cultivated in Japanese, Chinese, and even American cultures. Here in the United States, massive ginkgo trees can be spotted from a mile away. Their distinct leaf pattern is awe-inspiring and magical.

FACT

Ginkgos are nearly indestructible trees. After the atom bomb that was dropped on Hiroshima in 1945, there was nearly complete decimation of life. Six ginkgo trees survived the blast, although almost all other plants and animals were destroyed. A website documents the modern-day protection and historical significance of those trees that still stand today. For more information, go to *http://kwanten.home.xs4all.nl/ hiroshima.htm.*

Ginkgo Benefits

Ginkgo information is confusing for researchers because there are studies on both sides of the fence. Some discuss the great effectiveness of consuming the extract, and some suggest that there is no benefit whatsoever. The *Journal of Child and Adolescent Psychiatry and Psychotherapy* from Germany studied the effects of *Ginkgo biloba* extract on children with ADHD, and found that 240 mg a day resulted in positive effects. Ginkgo is therefore recommended as an alternative treatment for children with ADHD.

Ginkgo is a monoamine oxidase inhibitor (MAOI), meaning that those taking antidepressants such as SSRIs should not use or combine their medications with ginkgo. If you do, you could experience an increased risk of developing serotonin syndrome, which is not as fun as it sounds; it can be life-threatening in some cases. Serotonin syndrome causes symptoms that can range from shivering and diarrhea to fever and seizures. Milder forms may go away within a day of stopping the medications that cause symptoms. There are concerns over the side effects of taking ginkgo that sound similar to some prescription drugs, such as nausea, vomiting, headaches, and diarrhea. However, this shouldn't scare you away, as it's unlikely the effects would be experienced while taking a controlled supplemental dose.

A 2012 study looked at hospital and community health center subjects in Shanghai who complained about their memory, and gave them six months' worth of treatment with ginkgo. Using only about a 20 mg dose three times a day, the scores of the patients' logical memory and picture recognition increased significantly.

Here in the United States, you will find *Ginkgo biloba* as part of many different supplement stacks, ranging from brain health to memory enhancement and cognitive boosters. Long-term supplement trials, however, are almost non-existent to date.

A 2013 study in the *Public Library of Science* assessed the association between ginkgo supplementation and cognitive function over a 20-year period. They found that the cognitive function of the ginkgo supplementation group declined less rapidly than the group without treatment. Another group in the study used piracetam as their nootropic of choice, and found that this same beneficial effect was not attained. When compared to the piracetam and no treatment group, the ginkgo group had the only and most profound effect on preventing mental decline. The search terms "ginkgo" and "memory" in the U.S. National Library of Medicine reveals over 200 results for human trials, more than enough to verify the effectiveness and great potential for ginkgo to boost your brain.

Huperzine A

Massive trees and small plants both contain powerful chemicals that are capable of enhancing the function of your brain. *Huperzine serrata* meets that classification. It is a plant known as a firmoss that contains a nootropic compound called huperzine A. Huperzine A acts on the acetylcholine system and is an acetylcholinesterase inhibitor, giving it a powerful effect on cognitive function.

When you modify any neurotransmitter system, especially the cholinergic system, you may experience mild side effects such as nausea or diarrhea in the case of excess ingestion. This isn't likely to be the case if you are purchasing and supplementing with a product containing huperzine, otherwise they'd go out of business.

Acetylcholine inhibitors such as huperzine allow for an increase of acetylcholine in the brain, as it prevents the breakdown of neurotransmitters. Similar to the function of SSRIs, which keep the existing serotonin in the brain longer for a boost, huperzine allows for a greater accumulation of acetylcholine, which is able to significantly improve cognitive function.

Huperzine Research

Huperzine has been used before surgery requiring general anesthesia. Anesthesia is necessary for some operations, but the side effects and recovery time from anesthesia are some of its less desirable qualities. Administering huperzine before anesthesia, then comparing acetylcholine levels before and after the surgery requiring anesthesia, researchers found higher levels in those who were given huperzine, suggesting that cognitive recovery would be faster in that group. It should be said that it was administered intravenously in this case, which is not going to be your method.

In a trial run on subjects with mild to moderate dementia, 12 weeks of huperzine A supplementation significantly improved cognitive function, and no adverse effects were found. The control group without treatment did not have any improvement, throwing out the idea that someone could just magically heal their brain by chance. Huperzine effects are real and verified, and should be considered when developing your first nootropic stack.

Since the effects may not be felt immediately upon ingestion, combining huperzine with another more stimulatory compound such as low-dose caffeine found in matcha tea could give a great effect and mild boost to the brain and memory center. Since huperzine is also able to cross the blood-brain barrier, combining the naturally occurring L-Theanine with it can improve your symptoms of forgetfulness and memory trouble.

Relora

Relora is a patented and proprietary blend of two separate natural compounds designed for synergy. *Magnolia officinalis* is a tree native to China that has a highly aromatic bark used for its medicinal properties. The compounds found within magnolia bark act on the GABA system, leading to incredible anti-anxiety and mood-stabilizing effects. The other component of Relora is better known by its common name, the amur corktree.

It's widely known that stress, anxiety, insomnia, and excess body weight are linked together. The combination of these symptoms can diminish cognitive ability as well, and can lead to a snowball effect of misery in some cases. This is where Relora comes in.

Relora Effects

A 2008 study in *Nutrition Journal* found that overweight but otherwise healthy female adults who ate more in response to stressful situations were supplemented with 250 mg of Relora for 6 weeks. The supplement wasn't able to alleviate their long-term and pre-existing anxiety and depression, but their "transitory anxiety" was reduced, likely resulting in a reduction of stress eating.

Relora supplementation is not directly used to boost the brain, but rather to give the body relief from emotions that can sabotage cognitive function. If you are overwhelmed with stress and cope by consuming sugar or poor-quality caffeinated soda beverages, you are directly influencing your body's inflammatory load and your ability to think clearly.

By working on the underlying emotions causing poor lifestyle choices via supplementation, you may unlock a newfound sense of power over emotional eating and other poor choices made when you are stuck in a sympathetic fight-or-flight state.

CHAPTER 9

Mind-Enhancing Herbs

Herbs are used across the world for culinary, medicinal, and spiritual reasons. There are many different parts of herbs that can be used medicinally, such as leaves, roots, flowers, seeds, resin, and bark or fruit portions of the plant. Medicinal herbs contain phytochemicals, or "plant chemicals," that are capable of relieving depression and stress, boosting energy and cognitive function, or even causing pain relief and psychedelic states. Herbs have been used by ancient societies for over 8,000 years, as in the case of Peruvian people using cannabis and coca plants. In modern times, high-performing executives and athletes alike have sought out the use of herbs for enhancing performance.

Rhodiola rosea

One of the most popular and widely effective herbs is *Rhodiola rosea*, commonly referred to as golden root. This herb grows in cold, intense climates around the world and is historically used by Siberian people to help them adapt to such extreme temperatures. *Rhodiola rosea* was included in *De Materia Medica*, which translates to "on medical material," a pharmacopeia of herbs and medicines that was written by Roman physician Pedanius Dioscorides. This text dates between 50 and 70 AD, and is one of the most valuable medicinal texts in existence.

Rhodiola Benefits

Modern supplement companies market rhodiola as a mood and energy-boosting compound. It's great for reducing fatigue and increasing endurance. If you have a physical job or hobby such as construction, gardening, hiking, biking, swimming, etc., you may be very interested in rhodiola's benefits.

Siberians aren't the only ones who integrate rhodiola into their lifestyle. The Inuit people of Nunavik and Nunatsiavut in northeastern Canada regularly use rhodiola as a mental and physical rejuvenating agent. Whether the goal is to help adapt to the cold weather or to build up one's energy stores to hunt for hours on end, it's an important herb to these cultures.

FACT

Rhodiola is a mild but incredibly effective herb. If you're in the labor-related field, consider it an essential supplement for your arsenal. You'll be amazed at the mood and energy boost within a few weeks of consistent supplementation. Outperform your coworkers with ease and get that raise you deserve.

Rhodiola is typically found in alcohol extracts or capsule form, and generally contains 3 percent rosavins, which is the compound thought to be responsible for the antidepressant and anti-anxiety effects of the plant. In more recent studies, another compound found in rhodiola known as salidroside was found to be more active than rosavin. Salidroside is available in some rhodiola supplement formulations. It's best to seek out a combination of these nutrients, in a supplement that will most likely be labeled as 3 percent rosavins and 1 percent salidrosides.

Rhodiola is considered an adaptogenic herb, which allows it to be used with success in nearly any stressful situation. Adaptogenic herbs such as rhodiola allow a different perception of a stressful situation to exist. In a 2013 study by the *Journal of Strength and Conditioning Research* on the effects of rhodiola supplementation on endurance exercise performance (10-minute warm-up with a 6-mile time trial on a bicycle ergometer), researchers found that rhodiola ingestion significantly decreased heart rate during the warm-up and reduced how difficult the exercise seemed, which increased the performance.

In other words, rhodiola didn't directly alter the performance of the subjects, but it allowed them a sense of power over their workout, leading to reduced fatigue. This is the beauty that lies within adaptogenic herbs. When faced with a stressful or even dangerous situation, if you are taking rhodiola, you may have an increased ability to handle the situation rationally without panic or becoming paralyzed with other common reactions.

Depending on the person, rhodiola can be an acute or long-term supplement used to revitalize the nervous system and enhance the mood. For some reason, some may notice the first few doses if ingested in adequate amounts, while others feel no effect until regular supplementation for several weeks.

ALERT

The goal of adaptogenic herbs is different than most compounds. Adaptogens simply support the nervous system, mind, and body in a way that encourages a gentle but effective boost in nearly all aspects of performance. Adaptogens should be considered as part of a healthy diet regimen for anyone looking to perform their best and age gracefully without becoming overwhelmed by the stressors of modern life.

A 2012 study from *Phytotherapy Research* used *Rhodiola rosea* extract as a 4-week treatment protocol for subjects with life-stress symptoms. All tests showed clinically relevant improvements for stress symptoms and no adverse effects were found. The dose of 200 mg twice a day for four weeks is safe and effective.

Taking a Big Dose versus Spreading Them Out

The question with many supplements is whether you should take a consistent dose throughout the day or take one large dose at once. In the case of multivitamins, for example, it would be nearly impossible to obtain all of the necessary nutrients, micronutrients, minerals, and vitamins from one dose. Therefore, effective multivitamins should be taken throughout the day to give an adequate and steady stream of nutritional support.

However, herbs and cognitive boosters may be the opposite. Instead of taking rhodiola several times per day, it has been shown that it's best to take one good-sized dose near the beginning of your day to give the most effect. A study split subjects into two groups. One group that took 2 capsules of rhodiola after breakfast were compared to those that took 1 capsule after breakfast and 1 capsule after lunch. Even though they had the same dosage overall, the group that took all of their doses in one sitting after breakfast had more pronounced improvements, signifying that it's not the overall dose that matters, but how much you can get into the system at one time.

Try both methods of supplementation and see what's most helpful for you. A lot of people are too busy to keep up with taking different supplements at different times of the day, so be realistic with yourself and your schedule. Buying supplements for experimentation is only half the battle; actually remembering to take them consistently and in sufficient quantities is the most important part.

Call It Life Support

If you are over the age of 40, you should consider taking rhodiola. Since researchers and health care practitioners alike are beginning to view the mid-life crisis as more of a breakdown of normal hormonal and cognitive function, interventions to prevent or delay this occurrence should be of utmost importance. A 2008 journal entry in *World Psychiatry* states that chaotic changes in hormone levels, primarily associated with declining estradiol levels, may be one of the major factors in increased risk of depression, stress, and poor lifestyle choices. At the age of 40, you should still have plenty of energy and vitality to do outdoor activities and even compete in some athletic competitions with similarly aged individuals. For more information on this, see *www.ncbi.nlm.nih.gov/pmc/articles/PMC2559916*.

The aging process and stress that comes with more responsibilities can be aided by supplementing with rhodiola. Whether you're a stay-at-home dad who has a busy schedule juggling all of your kids' athletic calendars plus your own, or a stockbroker staring at three computer screens for 16 hours a day biting her nails, rhodiola may be your savior.

Ashwagandha

Withania somnifera, sometimes referred to as Indian ginseng, is an adaptogenic herb that has been used for over 4,000 years in India. It will be referred to by its common name ashwagandha throughout this section. The Latin name *somnifera* roughly translates to "sleep-inducing," although it can be used for energy production as well.

FACT

In general, the various forms of stress can deplete neurotransmitters, which results in deficiencies that can identify as symptoms of a poor and unfocused mood. Ashwagandha is capable of enhancing the catecholamine neurotransmitters, which include adrenaline and dopamine. Dopamine is responsible for personal drive and a healthy memory.

Ashwagandha Benefits

Cognitive impairment and bipolar disorder are linked and present a real issue for the millions of people who are affected by this disorder. A 2013 study from the *Journal of Clinical Psychiatry* took 60 subjects with bipolar disorder and enrolled them into an 8-week trial of using 500 mg of ashwagandha extract. Auditory-verbal working memory, reaction time, and social cognition were all improved in the supplement group without any major side effects.

Ashwagandha is a great supplement for those dealing with burnout or those struggling with adrenal fatigue. It provides a long-term rejuvenating effect on the body and supports the system as a whole. It can be taken in the morning for a steady flow of energy to the mind and body, and can also be taken again at night before bed to support deep, restful sleep. Many people who struggle with cognitive deficits also struggle with falling or staying asleep. Ashwagandha can be an incredible sleep aid that gives a mild afterglow effect the next morning.

FACT

Ashwagandha is unique. If you're taking it, you may not notice it until you stop taking it. The gentle and smooth boost that you've been riding suddenly disappears and you realize that rush-hour traffic is getting on your nerves more than usual. No one likes traffic, but consider it time to take your supplement again—you need it!

You may take 500 mg of ashwagandha extract before bed and notice that you sleep deeper than you do with melatonin supplementation, the typical recommendation by most people struggling with sleep issues. Melatonin presents withdrawal and down regulation effects while ashwagandha does not. After a deep night of sleep with ashwagandha, you can wake up feeling energetic and even euphoric. Colors, sights, and sounds may seem brighter and more pleasurable. This is likely due to the dopaminergic effects of ashwagandha.

When studying the effects on rats, similar positive results on memory and attention were found, and researchers concluded that ashwagandha deserves the categorization as both an adaptogen and a nootropic.

Bacopa monnieri

Bacopa is a genus of 70–100 aquatic plants that contains one of the most important herbs for brain-function on the planet. Specifically, *Bacopa monnieri*, sometimes called the herb of grace or brahmi, is a cognitive enhancer that has a long history in Ayurveda. You may recognize a pattern in that all of the herbs originating in Ayurvedic medicine are now becoming a hot topic for Americans seeking a healthier and natural alternative to prescription brain boosters.

The active chemical compounds present in this beautiful herb are known as bacosides. Quality bacopa supplements will label their extraction ratio or percentage of standardized bacosides to assure you that you're purchasing an efficacious product. Meta-analysis of controlled trials on bacopa extract found great potential at improving the speed of attention and memory recall in subjects.

At a dosage ranging from 300–450 mg of extract per day, bacopa can be a great standalone supplement or it can be safely combined with other herbs for an even greater effect. Combining bacopa with rhodiola results in a brighter mood, more energy, and improved cognitive function.

Bacopa has a unique ability to protect dopamine receptor dysfunction in the brain, which helps maintain your energy and drive. The memory center in the brain, the hippocampus, is at risk for toxicity from heavy metals, including aluminum. For example, those who have used mainstream deodorants and other aluminum-containing health care products are at risk of hippocampus deterioration. In fact, when cancerous breast tissue is biopsied, it is shown to have high levels of aluminum. This is likely due to the fact that the armpit rapidly absorbs anything that is applied. Luckily, bacopa is capable of protecting the hippocampus and may be a useful supplement if you have a history of using such health care products. Note that there are many safe, aluminum-free alternatives available at your local grocery store or on the Internet.

Panax ginseng

Ginseng is an incredible family of herbs that possesses various adaptogenic effects. *Panax ginseng* is one form that is well researched for the positive effects on rejuvenating the mind and body. The name *Panax* can be translated as "cure-all." Other forms of ginseng include American and Siberian ginseng, but they are not the same herb and each has different effects. Ginseng is now one of the most popular herbal medicines used nutraceutically, with an annual sale of over $200 million.

Yin and Yang

Since *Panax ginseng* use is rooted in Chinese culture, you should be familiar with the terms yin and yang and how they relate to herbal medicine.

Yin and yang are words to describe opposing yet complementary forces of nature. Yang refers to male, positive, and warm energy, while yin refers to female, negative, and cold energy. In traditional Chinese medicine, a balance of these two forces is what creates good health.

Chinese medicine has long used *Panax ginseng* as a general tonic or adaptogen to promote longevity and enhance bodily functions. It's been claimed to be effective at combating stress, fatigue, oxidants, cancer, and diabetes. One 2004 study in *Circulation* called "Modulating Angiogenesis: The Yin and the Yang in Ginseng," documents the ambiguity about the effects of ginseng and notes "the existence of opposing active principles in the extract," supporting the theory that ginseng possesses both yin and yang properties.

Ginseng Benefits

There is a lack of research into the cognitive and mood effects of repeated ginseng ingestion. A 2010 study in *Human Psychopharmacology* administered 200 and 400 mg doses to thirty volunteers for 8 days. The 200 mg dose slowed a fall in mood, but the 400 mg dose improved calmness and mental arithmetic, giving it a nootropic-like effect.

A similar study using American ginseng, which has a different nutrient profile than *Panax ginseng*, was tested and found to significantly improve working memory and cognitive function, too! If you're unable to source *Panax ginseng*, you can safely and effectively benefit from its similar species.

It's generally better to go for a natural compound to support your brain function, when possible. The synthetic nature rightfully concerns some people interested in improving their cognitive ability. A 2013 study in the *British Journal of Pharmacology* compared the two nutraceuticals, ginseng and bacopa, which have consistent acute and chronic cognitive effects, to that of the smart drug modafinil. It was found that ginseng and bacopa had greater effects for specific cognitive tests over that found in modafinil use. Nature wins again.

Autism rates have skyrocketed exponentially in recent years, characterized by significant impairment in social interaction and verbal and nonverbal communication. This often leads to psychopharmacological intervention in addition to psychobehavioral therapies, but benefits are limited by adverse side effects. *Panax ginseng* is considered comparable with piracetam, a nootropic effective in the treatment of autism. In a 2009 study in the *Journal of Dietary Supplements*, *Panax ginseng* produced improvement in patients with autism and should be considered at least as an add-on therapy modality. For more information, go to *www.ncbi.nlm.nih.gov/pubmed/22435515*.

Panax ginseng is not only effective for those seeking to boost cognitive power who are perfectly healthy, but in more serious cognitive deficits such as Parkinson's disease. Basically, it keeps you moving around and functioning better than you would without supplementing with it. If motivation and balance in a pill exists, *Panax ginseng* fits the bill.

Lemon Balm

Lemon balm is an herb in the mint family that is native to the Mediterranean and Central Asian regions of the world. It's used for culinary flavoring and is a popular plant for distillation for use in essential oil blends. It smells wonderful and has medicinal effects on the brain when consumed in supplemental form via capsules or herbal tea. Lemon balm acts on the GABA receptors, making it a great anti-stress remedy. Lemon balm also acts on the acetylcholine receptors, which is likely the reason for its nootropic effects.

Lemon balm has been cultivated in North America, but has escaped cultivation, allowing it to spread wild across the country. Generally, invasive species aren't a good thing for the native ecosystem, but lemon balm may be one non-native plant to smile at during your next hike in the woods.

Lemon Balm Benefits

A 2002 study in *Pharmacology, Biochemistry and Behavior* using lemon balm, referred to as *Melissa officinalis* in research, documents a trial of supplementing with 300 and 600 mg doses of lemon balm, examining its cognitive performance effects and the modulation of mood after being put through a stress simulation test. Like most supplements, the higher 600 mg dose ameliorated negative mood effects. Subjects reported calmness and showed a significant increase in the speed of mathematical processing. Being calm but focused is quite the perfect combination of effects for your next exam. You decide whether you want to reveal your secret weapon to your friends or not.

Most supplements that give a nootropic effect have an antioxidant capability. A 2011 study from *Toxicology and Industrial Health* wanted to determine the capability of a lemon balm infusion on radiology staff exposed to persistent low-dose radiation during work. Fifty-five radiology staff members were asked to drink lemon balm infusion prepared like a tea bag for 30 days. There was a significant improvement in glutathione peroxidase levels and a reduction in plasma DNA damage.

Glutathione is the master antioxidant in the body that, when low, can be linked to many diseases. Boosting your glutathione levels becomes more important as you age, since levels naturally slump. Consider lemon balm a great supplement for calming yourself down at the end of a long workday or before a tough meeting that usually spikes your nervous system into a mild panic. Consider lemon balm essential if you are exposed to radiation in your work, if you live near sources of radiation, or if you are in fear of a nuclear apocalypse.

Since it's hard to measure growth of brain cells in humans, rats are commonly used as subjects in studies. A 2011 study in *Neurochemical Research* found that lemon balm was capable of neurogenesis, the growth of brain cells. One can't become a genius by simply drinking lemon balm, but if you or someone you know has suffered from brain injury or other chronic forms of cognitive degeneration, using lemon balm in combination with other nootropics is a great way to prevent or slow further degradation.

Shankpushi

The Latin name *Convolvulus pluricaulis* isn't much harder to pronounce than the common name of this perennial herb. It is compared to morning glory, and all parts of the herb are known to possess therapeutic benefits. Use of this plant originates in Indian and Chinese medicine for chronic cough, sleeplessness, epilepsy, anxiety, and more. It also possesses anti-stress, anti-depressant, anti-anxiety, antioxidant, and even analgesic properties.

Shankpushi refers to use of the whole plant. There is a bit of controversy about using the name shankpushi, since other countries use different species and also refer to them as shankpushi. It's uncommon to find shankpushi in isolation in supplemental forms. It's more common to find shankpushi as an ingredient in herb blends.

There is one particular blend accurately called "Joy" by a company called Organic India. The combination of organic herbs bacopa, gotu kola, shankpushi, and ashwagandha create the most potent synergy for an adaptogenic, memory, happiness, and anti-stress formula available. If you try it, you may walk around smiling for a few hours.

Organic herbs are always preferred, since you can be assured that chemicals and other potential toxins are not present. Most companies are aware that the nature of herbs is to suck up heavy metals from the soil, and will frequently test and disclose the safety information regarding their herbs.

Gotu Kola

The last and no less valuable herb, gotu kola, is becoming popular in the Western world. It's been used historically as a wound-healing and blood-purifying herb, but recent research has identified cognitive enhancing and simultaneous antianxiety benefits. You may find gotu kola supplements labeled as Indian pennywort. It has been known in China as a "miracle elixir of life" for over 2,000 years.

Gotu kola is consumed as a leafy green in the east, commonly eaten with rice and curry. It is said to go well with vegetarian dishes. In Vietnam and Thailand, the gotu kola leaf is used for preparing a green refreshment drink, a great step up from the sugary green concoctions found in soda cans and energy drinks in the United States.

Gotu Kola Benefits

When applied topically, gotu kola increases the formation of collagen, the connective proteins that are responsible for healthy tissue. Trials for whether it provides a cognitive boost are lacking, but one 2008 study in *Journal of Ethnopharmacology* using gotu kola daily for two months found that elderly patients experienced an increase in working memory and mood. Mental clarity and reducing fatigue are some of the most notable effects of gotu kola.

Are you someone who startles easily? If someone pops up and tries to scare you or a loud unexpected noise happens, are you one to scream and hold your hand to your mouth? People who startle easily have a nervous system response that may be overactively engaged in the sympathetic mode.

As part of the anti-anxiety response that occurs when supplementing with gotu kola, it was found to be effective at reducing the acoustic startle response, a fancy name for being scared when a loud bang goes off. This isn't directly related to cognitive performance, but if you are needing to focus in a noisy environment for your job or other tasks, gotu kola may be helpful at calming the nervous system down enough for you to do so.

Moving Forward

You have just navigated through tens of thousands of years of ancient wisdom combined with decades of modern science to discover some of the most potent, effective, and valuable compounds and substances in existence. Take your time and start slowly with your experimentation. You can go bankrupt trying to buy one of everything. You'll find your favorite compounds in time.

There is no right or wrong place to start with your experimentation. You are a unique individual with a unique lifestyle. Searching the Internet for nootropic blends can be a good way to get an assortment of compounds for a good price, but it will be impossible to identify what is working well for you and what may be causing headaches or other side effects.

Adaptogens are the most accessible and widely beneficial compounds, so if you want direct guidance, start there. Eventually you can branch out to more specific compounds for boosting mental clarity, such as the synthetics and smart drugs. Enjoy yourself and understand that you are helping in progressing the future of natural medicine and your results should be spread as far and wide as possible.

Creating a Brain Stack

Stacking refers to combining nutrients, compounds, nootropics, or other supplements together to increase their effects or to attempt to balance out the neurotransmitters. For example, L-Theanine boosts GABA levels, which would result in a slightly calmer nervous system. If you were supplementing with L-Tyrosine, which can be too stimulating for some, you could combine L-Theanine and vinpocetine to boost memory power and balance out the stimulating effects of tyrosine.

If your goal is to enhance attention speed and increase brain power, you could use a more stimulating compound such as a low dose of caffeine (40 mg or so) and combine it with theanine, alpha-GPC, and vinpocetine to create a calm but alert state of the mind and body. This is the fun part about nootropics!

Depending on your unique biochemistry, your diet, your sleep quality, your stress levels, and your sensitivity to supplementation, you may need much more or less of an ingredient to satisfy your needs. Companies are experimenting with creating stacks that can be widely distributed to people who don't have the time or interest in researching various compounds to make their own stack.

Supplement Stack Building

Caffeine is addictive and can cause withdrawal effects. If a supplement has a high dose of caffeine (above 100 mg) it's probably because the other ingredients don't make you "feel anything" and they think you won't enjoy it otherwise. Many pre-workout supplements and some brain supplements contain high doses of caffeine to create a dependence and extreme boost of energy. The benefits of caffeine are short-lived and there are much better ways to boost your brain and body.

Some companies use proprietary blends on their supplement labels. Essentially, you'll see a list of ingredients but you will not know the dosage of each ingredient. There are a few reasons why companies do this. They either don't disclose the dosage to protect their formula, or because they are "fairy dusting," which means they are using a less than effective dose of a compound to save money, but they can still advertise it as containing that substance.

For example, *Cordyceps sinensis* can be considered an expensive compound to some, and companies may withhold their dosage by adding it in a blend of nutrients as opposed to specifically labeling a 200 mg dose. Just because a company uses proprietary blends doesn't mean they are trying to be sneaky, but asking more questions about the quality and efficacy of the dosages within is advised. Most consumers aren't this picky, but when you're trying to maintain an advantage over your peers in cognition and performance, details matter.

Some supplement manufacturers create patented versions of nutrients to make a profit, but also to ensure that an efficacious dose is administered.

If you see a trademarked supplement on an ingredient list, you can often assume that it is higher quality and that the dosage has been precisely calculated and researched. This is not always the case, but many supplement companies use at least a few of these types of ingredients to convince consumers of their quality and effectiveness.

Just because two supplements have the same ingredient doesn't mean the quality and effectiveness is the same. There can be differences in the effects and toxins present in a supplement if a mushroom was grown organically or with chemicals, for example. It would be rare for a company to purposely use chemicals in something grown for human consumption, but organic certification goes a long way in verifying that you're consuming a safer and generally more healthful form of a compound.

If you are not sure where to start, spending some time on *www.amazon.com* and seeking out these supplements can be a fun and helpful task. Reading reviews of others' experiences with them may provide a more realistic expectation and can help you determine your starting point. Since adaptogens can be beneficial for brain and body enhancement, they are a good place to start your research and experimentation. Combining an adaptogen with a brain-boosting fungus can give a great effect in a safe way.

CHAPTER 10

Breakfast

Mini Quiche

*These are a tasty treat for breakfast (or anytime!) and can be
made in bulk for easy mornings during the week.*

INGREDIENTS | SERVES 8

6 large eggs
3 ounces bacon
½ cup chopped broccoli
½ cup sliced mushrooms
½ cup diced onions
½ cup diced red peppers

1. Preheat oven to 325°F. Line muffin tin with 8 foil cups.

2. Whisk 6 eggs and set aside.

3. In a medium sauté pan over medium heat cook bacon until done, about 5–8 minutes. Drain on paper towels and chop into ½" pieces.

4. Spray a medium sauté pan with cooking spray. Sauté all remaining ingredients for 5 minutes.

5. Pour eggs into foil cups, filling each ⅔ of the way.

6. Add bacon and vegetables to each cup.

7. Bake 25 minutes or until golden brown.

Breakfast Salad

*Salad isn't just for lunch and dinner anymore. When you are trying to incorporate
more superfoods into your diet, salads should be round-the-clock meals.*

INGREDIENTS | SERVES 1

3 cups baby spinach leaves
2 large eggs, hard-boiled, peeled, and quartered
2 slices nitrate-free bacon, cooked and chopped
½ cup sliced cucumber
½ diced avocado
½ medium apple, sliced
½ medium lemon

1. Arrange spinach leaves on a plate and top with eggs and bacon.

2. Add cucumber, avocado, and apple slices to top of salad.

3. Squeeze fresh lemon juice over the salad. Serve immediately.

Bacon and Vegetable Omelet

Bacon and eggs are a breakfast tradition. Here they're combined with fresh summer squash, mushrooms, zucchini, and basil for a hearty and nutritious meal.

INGREDIENTS | SERVES 2

6 slices nitrate-free bacon, diced

1 medium yellow summer squash, chopped

1 cup mushrooms, sliced

1 medium zucchini, chopped

¼ cup fresh basil leaves, diced

2 tablespoons olive oil

8 large eggs, beaten

1. In a large sauté pan over medium heat, cook bacon until crispy, 5–8 minutes. Add the vegetables and basil to the pan and sauté until tender, approximately 5–8 minutes.

2. Heat olive oil in a second sauté pan over medium heat.

3. Cook eggs for 3 minutes on each side.

4. Place the vegetable and bacon mixture on one half of the eggs and fold over the other half to enclose the filling. Serve.

Protein Smoothie

This protein shake is a nutritious way to have a good meal on the go. You don't need to leave the house without breakfast anymore when you can make this fast, take-away breakfast.

INGREDIENTS | SERVES 1

2 tablespoons vanilla grass-fed whey protein powder

8 ounces no-sugar-added coconut water

1 tablespoon almond butter

⅛ teaspoon cinnamon

⅛ teaspoon nutmeg

Add all ingredients to a blender and blend until combined completely.

Protein Shakes

Protein shakes are the perfect way to give your body what it needs after exercise or a race event. They are quick and transportable, and they taste great!

Breakfast Bowl

This breakfast is a bit more exciting than the ordinary breakfast you might be used to, and is a great option if you're following the Paleo lifestyle. Nitrate-free, uncured bacon is a real treat.

INGREDIENTS | SERVES 1

2 tablespoons olive oil
½ cup diced uncured bacon
1 cup diced asparagus
2 large eggs

1. Heat olive oil in skillet over medium-high heat. Cook bacon and asparagus in skillet until asparagus is not quite tender, about 8–10 minutes. Remove to small bowl.

2. In the same skillet, cook eggs over easy (do not flip) about 5 minutes. Be sure that yolks are runny.

3. Place cooked eggs on top of bacon mixture.

4. Mix and serve.

Power-Packed Protein Shake

This shake will restore glycogen storage and provide your body with amino acids to rebuild torn tissue.

INGREDIENTS | SERVES 1

1 tablespoon coconut oil
8 ounces coconut water
2 tablespoons vanilla grass-fed whey protein powder

Add all ingredients to a blender and blend until combined completely.

Coconut Cacao Cookies

When you're craving a sweet breakfast, try these coconut cacao cookies. They are quick and satisfying.

INGREDIENTS | YIELDS 12–14 COOKIES

7 pitted dates
¾ cup almond flour
¼ cup coconut flour
½ cup shredded, unsweetened coconut
1 teaspoon coconut oil
2 tablespoons coconut milk
1 large egg
1 cup cacao nibs

Baking with Coconut

Coconut is a favorite when baking; its consistency provides a good base flour for any cookie or cake-like recipe. Try this coconut recipe when you are craving something sweet!

1. Preheat oven to 350°F.

2. Combine dates and unsweetened coconut in food processor and pulse until a crumb-like consistency is reached.

3. Pour mixture into a large mixing bowl and add remaining ingredients. Mix well with hands.

4. Form into patties and place on baking sheet sprayed with nonstick cooking spray.

5. Bake 22 minutes. Cool on a rack before serving.

Quick and Easy Protein Power Balls

This recipe is a perfect food for breakfast on the go. It is small, easily transported, and tastes great.

INGREDIENTS | YIELDS 8–10 BALLS

1 medium banana, peeled
2 tablespoons almond butter
2 tablespoons chocolate grass-fed whey protein powder

1. Mash banana and combine with almond butter and whey protein. If consistency is not thick, add more whey protein powder.

2. Using a tablespoon, scoop batter into palm and round into balls.

3. Store in refrigerator or freezer for later use.

Easy Pancakes

This pancake recipe is quick and easy and can be multiplied to make enough for an entire family. Once cooked, sprinkle the pancake with cinnamon or a small amount of agave nectar for an old-fashioned pancake taste.

INGREDIENTS | SERVES 1

1 medium banana, peeled
1 large egg
1 teaspoon nut butter of choice
2 teaspoons coconut oil

Bananas as Thickeners

Bananas can be a good replacement for flour. Bananas act as thickening agents in recipes that would normally be too fluid.

1. In a small bowl, mash banana with a fork.

2. In another bowl, beat egg and add to banana. Add nut butter and mix well.

3. Lightly coat medium frying pan or griddle with oil and preheat over medium heat. Pour entire pancake mixture onto preheated pan.

4. Cook until lightly brown on each side, about 2 minutes per side.

Poached Eggs

Poached eggs are very easy to make, but you must watch them or they will overcook. Time them exactly to get a perfect poached egg every time.

INGREDIENTS | SERVES 1

1 teaspoon apple cider vinegar
2 large eggs

1. Bring water to boil in a medium saucepan. Reduce heat to medium-low so that the water is simmering.

2. Add apple cider vinegar to water.

3. Crack and carefully slide eggs into the water.

4. Cook for exactly 3 minutes, remove with a slotted spoon, and serve.

Salmon Omelet with Asparagus and Dill

This omelet is full of omega-3 fatty acids. It is well seasoned and will surely become a breakfast staple.

INGREDIENTS | SERVES 2

2 tablespoons olive oil
¼ cup chopped green onions
1 cup trimmed and chopped asparagus
1 tablespoon chopped fresh dill
6 ounces salmon
6 large eggs, beaten

1. In a large skillet over medium heat, combine olive oil, green onions, asparagus, and fresh dill. Sauté until asparagus is soft, 5–10 minutes, and set aside.

2. In same skillet sauté salmon until flaky, about 10 minutes depending on thickness of steak. Set aside.

3. Wipe out the skillet and cook eggs on both sides until lightly browned, about 5 minutes each side.

4. Place salmon and asparagus mixture on half of egg, fold over, and serve.

Coconut Flour Pancakes

Cooking with wheat-free flours can be intimidating, but the sweet taste of coconut flour in these pancakes proves that even wheat-free pancakes can be delicious. You can replace the coconut oil with melted butter and the coconut milk with regular milk if you like.

INGREDIENTS | SERVES 3

2 whole large eggs
2 large egg whites
4 tablespoons coconut oil, divided
3 tablespoons coconut milk
1½ teaspoons maple syrup
1 teaspoon sea salt
3 tablespoons coconut flour
½ teaspoon wheat-free baking powder
1 teaspoon cinnamon
1 teaspoon allspice
⅓ cup ground flaxseed
1 teaspoon wheat-free vanilla extract

1. In a large bowl, using a wire whisk, mix together the eggs and egg whites, 3 tablespoons coconut oil, coconut milk, maple syrup, and salt.

2. Add the coconut flour and baking powder, whisking until thoroughly mixed. Add cinnamon, allspice, flaxseed, and vanilla. Stir to combine thoroughly.

3. Heat remaining tablespoon of coconut oil in a large skillet over medium heat.

4. Spoon 2–3 tablespoons of batter onto skillet, making pancakes about 3–4 inches in diameter. Cook 3–5 minutes, turning once.

Egg and Avocado Breakfast Burrito

Breakfast burritos are easy enough to make even on your busiest mornings.

INGREDIENTS | SERVES 4

6 large eggs
¼ cup shredded raw Cheddar cheese
⅓ cup milk
1 tablespoon olive oil
¼ medium yellow onion, peeled and finely chopped
½ medium green pepper, diced
2 avocados, peeled, pitted, and mashed
¼ teaspoon salt
½ teaspoon ground black pepper
4 corn or rice flour tortillas, warmed
⅔ cup crumbled goat cheese
¼ cup wheat-free salsa

1. In a medium bowl, beat together eggs, cheese, and milk until frothy.

2. Heat oil in a medium skillet over medium-high heat. Sauté onion and green pepper until onion is translucent, about 2–3 minutes.

3. Pour egg mixture into skillet and cook, stirring, until eggs are scrambled.

4. Season mashed avocados with salt and pepper.

5. Place tortillas one at a time in a separate skillet and cook until warm, about 2–3 minutes.

6. Spread equal amounts of avocado on one side of tortillas and layer with equal amounts of goat cheese and scrambled eggs. Roll up into burritos and serve immediately with salsa on the side.

Chocolate Chip–Zucchini Bread

You will never know that there are vegetables in this yummy bread or that it's wheat-free. It's a perfect way to sneak vegetables into your diet.

INGREDIENTS | SERVES 8

2 large eggs
½ cup coconut sugar
½ cup olive oil
½ cup unsweetened applesauce
1 tablespoon wheat-free vanilla extract
1 cup brown rice flour
½ cup almond flour
½ cup cornstarch
1 teaspoon xanthan gum
½ teaspoon wheat-free baking soda
¼ teaspoon wheat-free baking powder
½ teaspoon salt
1 tablespoon cinnamon
¼ teaspoon ground cloves
¼ teaspoon nutmeg
1½ cups fresh zucchini, shredded
½ cup dark chocolate chips, 70% or more cacao

1. Preheat oven to 350°F. Grease a 9" × 5" loaf pan with cooking spray.

2. In a large mixing bowl, beat together eggs, sugar, oil, and applesauce. Add the vanilla and mix well.

3. In a separate bowl, combine flours, cornstarch, xanthan gum, baking soda, baking powder, salt, cinnamon, cloves, and nutmeg.

4. Add dry ingredients to wet ingredients and mix well.

5. Add zucchini and chocolate chips and stir to combine.

6. Pour into the greased loaf pan and bake 60–70 minutes. Place a toothpick in center of bread and if it comes out clean, it's done.

Almond Butter–Raisin Cookies

These cookies are so easy to make. You can use other nut butters if you'd like. They also freeze very well.

INGREDIENTS | MAKES 24 COOKIES

1 cup unsalted almond butter, stirred well

¾ cup coconut sugar or sugar of your choice

1 large egg

½ teaspoon baking soda

¼ teaspoon sea salt (omit if almond butter is salted)

1 teaspoon wheat-free vanilla extract

½ teaspoon cinnamon

3 ounces raisins (you can also use dried cranberries, apricots, dates, cherries, or dried fruit of your choice)

1. Preheat oven to 350°F.

2. In a medium bowl, stir together all ingredients except raisins until blended.

3. Fold in raisins.

4. Drop dough by tablespoonfuls onto parchment-lined baking sheets. Bake 10–15 minutes or until lightly browned.

5. Let cool on baking sheets 5 minutes. Remove to a wire rack and let cool 15 more minutes.

Vegetable-Egg Scramble with Cheese

This light dish will be your favorite way to get your daily requirement of vegetables. If you don't have broccoli or tomatoes, use whatever vegetables you have in the house.

INGREDIENTS | SERVES 1

1 tablespoon olive oil
1 clove garlic, peeled and chopped
1 cup chopped broccoli
½ cup sliced grape tomatoes
3 large eggs
2 tablespoons chopped fresh basil
½ teaspoon sea salt
1 teaspoon oregano
1 tablespoon shredded Cheddar cheese

1. Heat the oil in a medium skillet over medium-high heat. Sauté the garlic 1 minute, then add the broccoli and tomatoes. Cook 2–3 minutes until broccoli is tender, but still crunchy.

2. Whisk eggs in a bowl until frothy.

3. Pour eggs into skillet and continue to mix thoroughly while eggs cook. Add basil, salt, oregano, and cheese, and cook for 3–4 minutes until eggs have light brown edges. Remove from heat and serve immediately.

Don't Pass on the Yolks, Folks

Are you using only egg whites? The yolks have a bad reputation, but they really are quite healthy. Yes, the yolks do contain cholesterol and fat, but moderate consumption of yolks will not put you at risk for the diseases they were once thought to have contributed to. The yolks also have a large amount of protein, calcium, and zinc, so don't be afraid to have some whole eggs, too!

Garlicky Vegetable Omelet

Delicious vegetables and garlic combine with fluffy eggs to make a simple, satisfying, and savory meal that will start any day off right. Protein-packed and rich in quality carbohydrates from the vegetables, this is a tasty way to get some valuable nutrition.

INGREDIENTS | SERVES 2

1 tablespoon butter
¼ cup chopped onions
¼ cup chopped mushrooms
2 tablespoons water
½ teaspoon garlic powder
¼ cup torn spinach leaves
5 large eggs (chicken or duck)

Gracious Garlic

A member of the lily flower family, garlic is a beautiful plant that can give your meal a tantalizing aroma and a unique flavor. Use just a single clove of this versatile plant to dress up tasteless dishes or to create a savory flavor.

1. Coat a small frying pan with butter and heat over medium heat.

2. Sauté onions for 1 minute. Add mushrooms and water, and continue sautéing until mushrooms are softened.

3. Sprinkle mixture with garlic powder and add the spinach leaves, stirring constantly.

4. Whisk together the eggs and pour the egg mixture over the sautéed vegetables.

5. Immediately begin pulling the outer edges into the center for one turn around the whole pan. Let the omelet set for 2 minutes.

6. Slide the spatula under the omelet, gently lifting the center from the pan. Once the omelet is balancing on the spatula, quickly flip the omelet over.

7. Continue cooking the omelet for another 3–5 minutes, or until no juices remain when pressed upon. Divide in half to serve.

Sweet Potato Hash Browns

The classic high-fat version of this breakfast staple gets a complete overhaul in this delicious hash brown recipe. By using fresh ingredients and butter, you can enjoy every last bite of these healthful hash browns.

INGREDIENTS | SERVES 6

1 tablespoon butter
3 medium sweet potatoes, shredded
1 small yellow onion, minced
1 large egg
2 tablespoons brown rice flour
1 teaspoon garlic powder
1 teaspoon salt
1 teaspoon freshly ground black pepper

1. Add butter to a large skillet and preheat over medium heat.

2. In a large mixing bowl, combine shredded potatoes, onion, egg, flour, and garlic powder and mix until thoroughly blended. Add salt and pepper to taste.

3. Form potato mixture into dense patties, using ½ cup of the mixture for each patty.

4. Add 2–3 hash brown patties at a time to the skillet. Cook 3–5 minutes, or until golden brown.

5. Flip patties and continue cooking until golden brown on both sides and completely cooked through.

Scrambled Egg Wrap

Perfect for a relaxing morning around the house, or as a breakfast to take with you in the car, these scrambled eggs are fragrant and full of flavor.

INGREDIENTS | SERVES 2

1 tablespoon butter
½ cup diced tomato
½ cup chopped spinach leaves
1 teaspoon garlic powder
1 teaspoon all-natural sea salt
1 teaspoon freshly ground black pepper
4 large eggs
2 tablespoons water
4 tablespoons full-fat plain yogurt
2 organic corn or rice flour tortillas

1. Coat a large skillet with butter and preheat over medium heat.

2. Sauté the tomato and spinach leaves with the garlic powder, salt, and pepper until spinach is wilted.

3. In a small mixing bowl, beat eggs and water. Pour eggs over vegetables and scramble until light and fluffy in consistency.

4. Spread 2 tablespoons of the yogurt down the center of each tortilla and top with the egg and vegetable mixture.

5. Wrap tightly and enjoy!

Mixed Vegetable Frittata

Packed with loads of protein from the eggs, and rich in healthy carbohydrates from all of the fresh vegetables, this is a great-tasting omelet. Customize it using your favorite vegetables.

INGREDIENTS | SERVES 4

1 tablespoon butter
½ cup chopped broccoli
½ cup mushrooms, cleaned and diced
½ cup chopped yellow pepper
¼ onion, chopped finely
12 large eggs
1 tablespoon garlic powder
1 teaspoon all-natural sea salt
2 teaspoons freshly ground black pepper

1. Preheat oven to 350°F. Coat a large oven-safe skillet with butter, and preheat over medium heat.

2. Combine broccoli, mushrooms, yellow pepper, and onion in the skillet with water and cook until tender, but not soft.

3. Whisk together eggs, garlic powder, salt, and black pepper and pour over veggie mixture.

4. Cook until the center begins to shake and bubble from the heat (about 3–4 minutes). Remove from heat and place in preheated oven for 15 minutes, or until center is set and an inserted fork comes out clean.

Turkey, Egg, and Hash Brown Bake

*You can beat any craving for a hearty, healthy breakfast with this satisfying dish.
Combining delicious ground turkey breast and hash brown potatoes in a one-pot dish,
this is a great meal for breakfast, brunch, or anytime you need a pick-me-up.*

INGREDIENTS | SERVES 16

1 tablespoon butter
1 pound ground turkey breast, browned
1 pound shredded sweet potatoes
12 large eggs
2 teaspoons all-natural sea salt
2 teaspoons freshly ground black pepper
1 teaspoon cayenne pepper

The Power of Egg Yolks

Egg yolks are one of the most nutrient-dense foods available. Egg yolks contain the essential vitamins and minerals that, when combined with other protein-rich foods, help the body's systems run efficiently for energy and recovery.

1. Preheat oven to 375°F.

2. Coat a 9" × 13" glass casserole dish with butter.

3. Combine ground turkey breast, potatoes, and eggs thoroughly.

4. Season with salt, black pepper, and cayenne.

5. Pour mixture into baking dish and let settle completely.

6. Bake for 30–40 minutes, or until top is golden and firm and inserted fork comes out clean.

Asparagus and Leek Frittata

A 4" or 5" cast-iron skillet works perfectly for this dish. Smaller skillets may be harder to find, but they're great for single servings and for when you just need to make a small amount of food.

INGREDIENTS | SERVES 1

1 stalk cooked asparagus, chopped

1 teaspoon unsalted butter

¼ cup chopped leeks

2 large eggs

2 tablespoons shredded raw and/or organic Parmesan cheese

2 tablespoons shredded Gruyère

1 teaspoon minced chives

¼ teaspoon salt

¼ teaspoon ground black pepper

Frittatas: An Economical Dish

Frittatas are the perfect way to use up small amounts of leftovers. A handful of leftover chicken, or any leftover vegetable can be substituted in this recipe. Just make sure the filling is warm when the eggs are added. Frittatas are almost always served well done, or firm.

1. Steam the piece of asparagus if it isn't already cooked. Place a seasoned cast-iron skillet over medium heat. Once it is warm add the butter and the leeks. Cook the leeks slowly and stir frequently for 8–10 minutes. Add the asparagus to the skillet.

2. Turn on the broiler. In a separate bowl, whisk together the eggs, cheeses, chives, salt, and pepper. Once the leeks are soft and the asparagus is warmed, pour the egg mixture into the skillet. Let the eggs cook for 5–6 minutes without stirring.

3. Once the bottom and sides of the eggs are firm, place the skillet under the broiler about 4" from the heat. Let the frittata cook until the top of the eggs are lightly browned, about 4–5 minutes.

4. Remove the pan from the oven and while it is still hot, run a thin knife along the edges of the skillet to loosen the frittata. Slide the frittata onto a plate and serve immediately.

Fresh Mushroom Scramble

Simple and fresh ingredients come together to create this tasty and satisfying breakfast scramble. If you'd like it to be dairy-free, simply omit the milk. The consistency of the eggs will change just a bit.

INGREDIENTS | SERVES 4

10 large eggs

2 tablespoons milk

¼ teaspoon salt

¼ teaspoon ground black pepper

2 tablespoons organic Worcestershire sauce

2 small cloves garlic, crushed

2 teaspoons butter, melted

2 large fresh mushrooms, washed and stemmed

2 tablespoons chopped parsley

1. Lightly whisk the eggs in a large bowl with the milk until combined. Season with salt and pepper.

2. Combine the Worcestershire sauce, garlic, and melted butter. Brush the mushrooms lightly with the Worcestershire sauce mixture, then grill or broil on medium heat for 5–7 minutes or until soft. Remove and keep warm.

3. Heat a large nonstick frying pan and add the egg mixture, scraping the bottom gently with a flat plastic spatula to cook evenly. Cook until the egg is just set.

4. To serve, divide the scrambled eggs and mushrooms among four serving plates. Sprinkle the eggs with the chopped parsley. Serve immediately.

Spinach Omelet

The Parmesan cheese enhances the flavor of this omelet. The harmony of spinach and eggs makes this omelet highly nutritious but also elegant enough to serve to guests at your next brunch.

INGREDIENTS | SERVES 6

1 (10-ounce) package frozen chopped spinach, thawed and undrained

3 tablespoons bone broth

1 clove garlic, crushed

¼ teaspoon ground black pepper

¼ cup grated raw and/or organic Parmesan cheese

10 large eggs

2 tablespoons water

2 teaspoons butter, divided

Spinach Rating

Spinach is a great source of vitamins A and C, and it has lots of minerals, iron, potassium, and beta-carotene. Spinach has a high calcium count as well; however, spinach contains substances called "oxalates" which stop calcium absorption in extreme cases of overconsumption.

1. Combine spinach, broth, garlic, and pepper in a small saucepan; cover and simmer 20 minutes. Stir in Parmesan cheese; cook 1 minute or until cheese is melted, stirring constantly. Set aside.

2. Combine eggs and water; beat lightly. Coat a 10" omelet pan or heavy skillet with cooking spray; add 1 teaspoon butter. Place pan over medium heat until just hot enough to sizzle a drop of water.

3. Pour half of egg mixture into pan. As mixture starts to cook, gently lift edges of omelet with a spatula and tilt pan so uncooked portion flows underneath.

4. As mixture begins to set, spread half the spinach mixture over half the omelet. Loosen omelet with a spatula; fold in half and slide onto a warm serving platter.

5. Repeat procedure with remaining ingredients. Divide omelets evenly to serve.

Spicy Sausage and Venison Brunch Dish

If your butcher makes game breakfast sausage, then just use it for this recipe. Or use ground game and spice it up with fennel, red pepper flakes, and assorted herbs like oregano and basil. This casserole is easy to assemble at the last minute and holds well on a buffet. Oh! It's delicious, too.

INGREDIENTS | SERVES 8

1 tablespoon butter

½ pound ground venison

½ pound spicy breakfast sausage

¼ teaspoon salt

¼ teaspoon freshly ground black pepper

2 (4-ounce) green chilies, chopped

1 cup organic shredded Monterey jack cheese

12 large eggs

1½ cups organic raw whole milk

Wheat-free salsa and chopped scallions, to garnish

1. Preheat oven to 350°F. Coat a 9" × 13" glass casserole dish with butter.

2. Brown meat in a large skillet over medium-high heat. Place evenly in the baking dish. Season with salt and pepper. Sprinkle green chilies and cheese evenly over the meat.

3. With the back of a spoon, slightly hollow 12 places for the eggs (away from the edge of the baking dish). Break eggs into the indentations and lightly break yolks with a fork. Pour milk over all ingredients and bake for about 30–40 minutes, just until set.

4. Serve with salsa and chopped scallions on the side.

Olive Oil Smashed Potatoes

Place 4–6 potatoes, peeled or not, in a saucepan and cover with water. Cook over high heat for 20–25 minutes. When potatoes are fork tender, drain the water well. Smash the potatoes with a masher, just a couple of times. Drizzle with olive oil and sprinkle with salt and pepper to taste. Serve hot and lumpy.

Sweet Potato Pancakes

You'll never look at pancakes the same way again once you taste this sweet potato variety! Sweet, smooth, and flavorful, this healthier option outdoes the refined favorite in every aspect.

INGREDIENTS | SERVES 10

1 tablespoon butter
1 cup sweet potato purée
1 cup full-fat plain Greek yogurt
1 cup unsweetened applesauce
4 large eggs
2 teaspoons vanilla extract
2 tablespoons organic maple syrup
¼ cup rice flour
1 teaspoon baking powder
1 teaspoon pumpkin pie spice
1 teaspoon organic cinnamon

1. Coat a nonstick skillet with butter and place over medium heat.

2. Combine remaining ingredients and mix well.

3. Scoop the batter onto the preheated skillet, using approximately ½ cup of batter per pancake.

4. Cook 2–3 minutes on each side, or until golden brown. Remove from heat and plate immediately. Serve with your favorite egg dish on the side.

No Vitamin A Supplement Needed

Sweet potatoes are beautiful, naturally sweet versions of the much-loved potato. Packed with lycopene and carotenoids, these amazing spuds are also abundant in vitamin A. Amazingly, just one single sweet potato boasts more than two-and-a-half times the daily recommended amount of vitamin A. Just one sweet potato can reduce inflammation, protect against free radical damage, and supply a great amount of vitamin A.

CHAPTER 11

Lunch

Avocado Chicken Salad

In addition to being a quick, delicious lunchtime treat, this recipe works well as a party salad if you double or triple the ingredients. You can serve it in lettuce cups for a meal or in small cups with spoons as an appetizer.

INGREDIENTS | SERVES 3

3 avocados, pitted and peeled

2 boneless, skinless chicken breasts, cooked and shredded

½ medium red onion, chopped

1 large tomato, chopped

¼ cup chopped cilantro

Juice of 1 large lime

1. In a medium bowl, mash avocados. Add chicken and mix well.

2. Add onion, tomato, cilantro, and lime juice to the avocado and chicken mixture. Mix well and serve.

Easy Slow Cooker Pork Tenderloin

Slow cooker meals are a great way to cook for your family. Large quantities can be thrown into the cooker hours in advance. Most leftovers can be easily frozen for future meals.

INGREDIENTS | SERVES 4

1 pound lean pork loin, whole

1 (28-ounce) can diced tomatoes, no salt added

3 medium zucchinis, diced

4 cups cauliflower florets

2 tablespoons chopped fresh basil

1 clove garlic, peeled and chopped

1. Combine all ingredients in slow cooker.

2. Cook on low 6–7 hours.

3. Before serving, remove tenderloin from the slow cooker and place on a platter, tented with foil, to rest 5–10 minutes. Slice and serve with your favorite sides.

Chipotle Pulled Pork

This pulled pork recipe has super flavors. Adjust the spices as needed to kick it up a notch or cool it down. Either way, this recipe is sure to please the entire family.

INGREDIENTS | SERVES 8

2½ pounds pork loin

1 large onion, peeled and chopped

1 (16-ounce) can unsalted organic tomato paste

3 tablespoons olive oil

2 cups lemon juice

½ cup unsalted beef broth

4 cloves garlic, peeled

¼ teaspoon cayenne pepper

½ teaspoon paprika

2 teaspoons chipotle chili powder

1 teaspoon thyme

1 teaspoon cumin

1. Combine all ingredients in a slow cooker.

2. Cook on low 5 hours or until meat is softened completely.

3. Once cooled, shred with fork and serve.

Chicken Enchiladas

If you have been craving a Mexican feast, try this spicy carb-free version of traditional enchiladas. Wrapping the filling in collard greens ups the flavor and provides an extra burst of vitamins!

INGREDIENTS | SERVES 8

2 tablespoons olive oil

2 pounds boneless, skinless chicken breast, cut in 1" cubes

4 cloves garlic, peeled and minced

½ cup finely chopped onion

2 cups chopped tomatoes

1 teaspoon ground cumin

1 teaspoon chili powder

½ cup fresh cilantro

Juice from 2 medium limes

1 (10-ounce) package frozen chopped spinach, thawed and drained

8 collard green leaves

1. Heat olive oil in a medium skillet over medium heat. Sauté chicken, garlic, and onion in the hot oil until thoroughly cooked, about 10 minutes.

2. Add tomatoes, cumin, chili powder, cilantro, and lime juice and simmer 5 minutes.

3. Add spinach and simmer 5 more minutes. Remove from heat.

4. In a separate pan, quickly steam collard greens to soften, about 3 minutes.

5. Wrap chicken mixture in collard greens and serve.

Turkey Meatballs

This is a simple and delicious meatball recipe with some basic additions. You can substitute any type of ground meat you prefer: bison, beef, chicken, or pork. Flaxseed meal can replace the almond meal as well.

INGREDIENTS | SERVES 8

2 pounds (93% lean) ground turkey

1 cup almond meal

2 large eggs

5 scallions, chopped

1 medium red bell pepper, diced

2 cloves garlic, peeled and minced

1 tablespoon dried basil

1 tablespoon dried oregano

2 tablespoons olive oil

1. Preheat oven to 400°F.

2. Combine all ingredients except olive oil in a large bowl. Mix well.

3. Add olive oil to turkey mixture and mix well.

4. Form turkey mixture into 24 meatballs and place in 2 rimmed baking pans.

5. Bake 20 minutes.

Higher Fat Ground Meats

Although most people make sure to buy the lowest fat ground meat, it is more beneficial to buy fattier ground meat when it is from grass-fed or barn-roaming animals. This meat is lower in saturated fat than most commercial ground meat, and the fat profiles favor the omega-3 fatty acids to fight inflammation and heart disease in your body.

Wheat-Free "Spaghetti"

This is a great alternative to traditional pasta. Serve with sauce and Turkey Meatballs (see recipe in this chapter) for a healthier take on Grandma's spaghetti and meatball recipe!

INGREDIENTS | SERVES 4

1 large spaghetti squash

Pasta Alternative

Spaghetti squash is a fantastic carbohydrate source for all you pasta addicts out there. This squash looks like spaghetti when the meat is peeled from the skin. It has the relative texture of pasta. And, most importantly, it is quite filling.

1. Preheat oven to 350°F.

2. Cut squash in half lengthwise.

3. Place cut-side down in baking dish with ¼" water.

4. Cook 30 minutes, then turn over and cook until soft all the way through when pierced with fork, approximately 10 minutes.

5. Shred with fork and serve.

Grilled Jerk Chicken

This marinated chicken dish is great to cook in large quantities for eating throughout the week. It is a fantastic summer dish to make outside on the grill.

INGREDIENTS | SERVES 4

5 cloves garlic, peeled and chopped
1 teaspoon ginger powder
1 teaspoon dried thyme
1 teaspoon ground paprika
1 teaspoon ground cinnamon
½ teaspoon ground allspice
½ cup lemon juice
½ cup red wine
4 boneless, skinless chicken breasts

1. Combine garlic, ginger, thyme, paprika, cinnamon, allspice, lemon juice, and red wine in a large bowl.

2. Add chicken and marinate for at least 5 hours in refrigerator.

3. Prepare a charcoal or gas grill.

4. Remove chicken from marinade and wrap in aluminum foil. Place foil packets on preheated grill and cook 12 minutes.

5. Remove chicken from aluminum foil and grill 5 minutes.

Pecan-Crusted Chicken

This pecan crust recipe is quite versatile. It works for fish as well as chicken, and other nuts can be substituted for different flavors.

INGREDIENTS | SERVES 4

1 cup finely chopped pecans
2 large eggs, beaten
4 boneless, skinless chicken breasts

Toasting Nuts for Fresher Flavor and Crispness

When serving nuts, whether on a salad, in a dish, or as a snack, toasting them brings out their delicious flavors and aromas. To wake the natural flavor of the nuts, heat them on the stovetop or in the oven for a few minutes. For the stovetop, spread nuts in a dry skillet, and heat over a medium flame until their natural oils come to the surface. For the oven, spread the nuts in a single layer on a baking sheet, and toast for 5–10 minutes at 350°F, until the oils are visible. Cool nuts before serving.

1. Preheat oven to 350°F.

2. Place chopped nuts in a shallow bowl and eggs in a separate shallow bowl.

3. Dip each chicken breast in egg and then in nuts. Place coated chicken breasts in a shallow baking dish.

4. Bake for 25 minutes.

Savory Beef Stew

This recipe was adapted from a traditional beef stew recipe. You will be surprised at how good this really tastes. Try adding sliced carrots, parsnips, or celery for extra flavor and vitamins.

INGREDIENTS | SERVES 10

¼ cup almond flour
½ teaspoon nutmeg
1 teaspoon cinnamon
½ teaspoon allspice
½ teaspoon ground black pepper
2 pounds chuck steak, cubed
2 tablespoons olive oil
2 medium onions, peeled and chopped
½ cup red wine
2 pounds button mushrooms, quartered
1 (14-ounce) can organic beef broth, unsalted
½ cup water

Alcohol in Cooking

Even if you don't drink, you may find it acceptable to use alcohol while cooking, since most of the alcohol is burned off. This is a nice way to bring some depth of flavor to your dish.

1. Combine almond flour, nutmeg, cinnamon, allspice, and pepper in a plastic bag.

2. Add chuck steak to plastic bag and shake to coat evenly.

3. Heat olive oil in a large skillet over medium-high heat.

4. Sear steak quickly in skillet 1–2 minutes each side. Remove from skillet and place in slow cooker.

5. Using the same skillet over medium heat, cook onion 8 minutes.

6. Add red wine to the skillet and cook 5 more minutes, until the onions are browned.

7. Add mushrooms, broth, and water to slow cooker. Cook at least 5 hours on low heat in slow cooker.

Roasted Pork Tenderloin

This pork tenderloin recipe will melt in your mouth and fill your kitchen with heavenly aromas. Serve leftovers sliced thin on a bed of crunchy romaine for lunch the next day.

INGREDIENTS | SERVES 6

Juice of 1 large orange
3 tablespoons lime juice
2 tablespoons red wine
10 whole cloves garlic, peeled
1 teaspoon dried thyme
¼ teaspoon freshly ground black pepper
2½ pounds pork loin

1. Combine juices, wine, garlic, thyme, and pepper in a large zip-top plastic bag.

2. Add pork to the bag and seal. Marinate at least 2 hours in refrigerator.

3. Preheat oven to 350°F. Remove pork from marinade and place in a shallow baking pan.

4. Cook 30 minutes or until the internal temperature reaches 165°F.

5. Remove from baking pan and let pork sit 5 minutes before carving.

Chipotle-Lime Mashed Sweet Potato

Sweet potatoes are a great post-workout food. These Chipotle-Lime Mashed Sweet Potatoes will be a favorite at any family table. Try serving with Roasted Pork Tenderloin (see recipe in this chapter) for a lunch that will power you through the rest of your day.

INGREDIENTS | SERVES 10

3 pounds sweet potatoes, peeled and cubed
1½ tablespoons coconut oil
1¼ teaspoons chipotle powder
Juice from ½ large lime

1. Steam the sweet potato cubes until soft, approximately 5–8 minutes. Transfer to a large bowl.

2. In a small saucepan, heat coconut oil and whisk in the chipotle powder and lime juice.

3. Pour the mixture into the bowl with the sweet potato cubes and mash with fork or potato masher.

Alternatives to Sweet Potatoes

If you don't like sweet potatoes, you can easily substitute some lower glycemic-load vegetables such as rutabagas, turnips, or beets. Cauliflower makes a great fake "mashed potato" substitute.

Coconut-Crusted Chicken

This is an easy way to add some flavor and crunch to chicken, and can be easily adapted to use on firm fish and shrimp. It is also a great way for little kids (and adults!) to enjoy eating with their hands.

INGREDIENTS | SERVES 8

1 cup ground almond meal
2 large eggs
2 teaspoons ground black pepper
1 tablespoon Italian seasoning
1 cup unsweetened coconut flakes
½ cup flaxseed meal
16 chicken tenderloins
4 tablespoons coconut oil

1. Pour almond meal into a shallow bowl. In another bowl, whisk eggs, pepper, and Italian seasoning. In a third bowl, combine coconut flakes with flaxseed meal.

2. Coat chicken pieces with the almond meal.

3. Transfer chicken to the egg mixture, then coat with coconut mixture.

4. Heat coconut oil in a large nonstick skillet over medium-high heat.

5. Pan-fry tenderloins until cooked through, approximately 5 minutes on each side, depending on thickness of chicken.

Comforting Chicken Soup

The major advantage of this soup is that it will be much lower in sodium than other canned chicken soups. The only limit is your imagination. Each time you make it, substitute different vegetables and seasonings to tantalize your taste buds.

INGREDIENTS | SERVES 6

5–6 pounds chicken (including giblets), cleaned, trimmed, and quartered

12 cups water

¼ bunch parsley, chopped

2 medium carrots, peeled and chopped

2 stalks celery, chopped

4 large yellow onions, peeled and chopped

¼ teaspoon freshly cracked black pepper

¼ teaspoon kosher salt

1. Place chicken and giblets in a stockpot, add water, and bring to a boil. Reduce heat to a simmer and skim off all foam.

2. Add all the remaining ingredients and simmer uncovered about 3 hours.

3. Remove chicken and giblets from the stockpot; discard giblets. Remove meat from bones, discard bones, and return meat to broth; serve.

Don't Cry over Cut Onions

The sulfur in onions can cause the tears to flow. To avoid teary eyes, peel onions under cold water to wash away the volatile sulfur compounds. Onions are worth it, since they have anti-inflammatory effects on the joints.

Grilled Turkey Tenders with Citrus Butter

If getting kids or the uninitiated game eater to try something they will love, this is it. Similar to grilled chicken fingers but with much more flavor, guests will find them delightful. This recipe also works well by cutting turkey breast meat into 1"-thick strips.

INGREDIENTS | SERVES 4

4 turkey tenderloins
6 tablespoons unsalted butter
Zest and juice of 1 lemon
½ teaspoon freshly ground black pepper
½ teaspoon hot sauce
½ teaspoon sea salt

Wild Turkey Tenderloins

Wild turkey is delicious. Its meat is sweet and more textured than farm-raised varieties. The tenderloin is the small strip of turkey breast meat closest to the bone. It is the most sweet and tender piece of meat on the whole turkey.

1. Prepare a hot fire in a grill. Rinse and dry turkey tenderloins. Place on a plate and set aside.

2. In a small saucepan, melt the butter over low heat and add the lemon, pepper, hot sauce, and salt. Brush butter mixture on both sides of turkey strips.

3. Place turkey tenderloins over the hot fire and grill for about 3 minutes on each side, brushing with additional citrus butter as needed. Turkey tenderloins should register 170°F for well-done.

Grillpan Salmon Caesar Salad

Adapt this Caesar salad recipe for the fish or meat of your choice.
Or serve it as a side salad without the meat.

INGREDIENTS | SERVES 4

4 (6-ounce) salmon fillets, ¾" thick

1 tablespoon olive oil

1 teaspoon seasoned pepper

5 tablespoons full-fat plain Greek yogurt

2 teaspoons anchovy paste

1 clove garlic, minced

1 teaspoon Dijon mustard

1 tablespoon lemon juice

¼ teaspoon salt

¼ teaspoon ground black pepper

1 head romaine lettuce, cleaned and torn

⅓ cup freshly grated Romano cheese

Are Salmon Freshwater Fish?

Yes, even though most species spend their lives in saltwater oceans. They are born in freshwater streams and immediately make haste for the ocean. Then, when ready to spawn, they return to almost the exact spot where they were born. This process of returning to freshwater streams to spawn tags salmon and char with the term *anadromous*.

1. Rinse salmon fillets and pat dry. Place on a plate and lightly coat with olive oil and seasoned pepper. Set aside.

2. To make dressing, combine the yogurt, anchovy paste, garlic, mustard, and lemon juice in a bowl and stir to blend. Taste and add salt and pepper to your liking. Set aside.

3. Preheat a grill pan or griddle over high heat. When hot, place salmon fillets on the pan. Cook for about 4 minutes per side. Remove from pan.

4. Place the lettuce in a large bowl. Toss with dressing to lightly coat the lettuce. Add the cheese and toss again.

5. Portion out ¼ of the lettuce on each of four plates. Top each with a salmon fillet.

Fall-off-the-Bone Duck

Every shred of meat can be eaten on Fall-off-the-Bone Duck. The bones pick clean. Use the bits of meat for any of your favorite soup or salad recipes. This recipe calls for 6–7 pounds of duck to be cooked, so it will either serve 8 people for a luncheon or you'll have scrumptious leftovers for another meal.

INGREDIENTS | SERVES 8

3 mallard ducks, or the equivalent of 6–7 pounds of duck

3 tablespoons salt

Freshly ground black pepper, to taste

2 medium apples, quartered

¼ cup raw honey

¼ cup sherry

1 tablespoon Worcestershire sauce

2 tablespoons butter

2 tablespoons almond flour

Freezing Ducks

Vacuum-seal freezer machines and bags cost a little over $100 and are the best for maintaining game in the freezer. Less costly, but also effective, is to wrap each duck in a 12" × 18" piece of plastic-coated freezer paper. Label dates on packages with a felt tip pen. Place 1 or 2 wrapped ducks in a resealable plastic freezer bag with as little air as possible. They will keep, frozen, for almost a year.

1. Place ducks in a large stockpot and cover with water. Add salt, pepper, apples, and bring to a boil. Cook for 45 minutes. Remove from water and place ducks in a large roasting pan.

2. Preheat oven to 375°F. Combine honey, sherry, and Worcestershire. Baste duck with sauce and place in oven for 30 minutes, uncovered.

3. Liberally baste again and add water to pan to prevent duck from sticking. Cover the pan tightly with a lid or cover tightly with heavy-duty foil.

4. Lower heat to 275°F. Roast for 2½–3 hours more, depending on size of ducks, basting every 30 minutes. Add water to bottom of pan if dry. Ducks are done when leg joint falls apart.

5. To make gravy, add 2 tablespoons butter and 2 tablespoons flour to pan juices and cook until slightly thickened.

Coconut and Basil Chicken

Even if you don't like spicy food, keep the jalapeño for its flavor. To significantly reduce the heat in this dish, cut away the jalapeño's seeds and white veins, which contain most of the heat.

INGREDIENTS | SERVES 4

1 scallion, chopped with white and green separated

2" piece ginger, peeled and cut into matchsticks

1 cup coconut milk

1 cup Thai basil leaves

3 cloves garlic

2 teaspoons raw honey

1 teaspoon fish sauce

½ pound boneless, skinless chicken breast or thighs

¼ teaspoon salt

½ teaspoon ground black pepper

1 tablespoon olive oil

1 jalapeño pepper, seeded and thinly sliced

½ cup chopped cilantro, for garnish

2 tablespoons toasted coconut for garnish

2 lime slices for garnish

4 cups cooked brown rice

1. Combine the scallion, ginger, coconut milk, basil, garlic, honey, and fish sauce in a blender and purée until smooth.

2. Remove any fat or skin from the chicken, cut the meat into 1" cubes, and sprinkle the chicken with salt and pepper.

3. Place a cast-iron skillet over medium-high heat and when it is warm, add the olive oil. Add the chicken. Cook for 3 minutes on each side, or until lightly browned. Reduce heat to medium-low.

4. Pour the coconut sauce and jalapeños over the chicken. Cover and cook for 8–10 minutes until the sauce just starts to bubble. Once the chicken is firm and no longer pink in the middle, it is ready to serve with the garnishes over cooked rice.

Garnishing Asian Dishes

People from many Asian cultures don't consider a meal complete without garnishes, which differ from cuisine to cuisine. This dish takes its influence from Thai cuisine and many Thai recipes are served with lime wedges, soy sauce, toasted coconut, chopped cilantro, or a spicy pepper sauce.

Ground Beef Tacos

You can use organic corn or rice tortillas in this recipe. Rice tortillas are soft and corn tortillas can be steamed lightly to soften them or fried to make them crunchy.

INGREDIENTS | MAKES 16 TACOS

1 tablespoon butter
1 medium onion, chopped
2 jalapeños, minced
3 cloves garlic, minced
1 tablespoon chili powder
1 tablespoon dried oregano
¼ teaspoon cayenne pepper
1 teaspoon salt
¼ teaspoon ground black pepper
2 pounds ground beef
16 small tortillas or taco shells
Wheat-free salsa, for garnish
Organic shredded cheese, for garnish
Chopped tomatoes, for garnish
Shredded leafy greens, for garnish
2 limes cut into wedges

1. Place a skillet over medium heat. Once it is warm add the butter, onion, and jalapeños. Sauté 5–7 minutes. Add the garlic and stir frequently for 2–3 minutes. Add the chili powder, oregano, cayenne, salt, and pepper and toss to combine.

2. Reduce the heat to low. Crumble the ground beef over the skillet and stir to cook. Once the outside of the meat is brown, cover the skillet with a lid and cook for 10 minutes.

3. Drain off the grease and discard.

4. Serve with warmed tortillas and top with salsa, cheese, tomatoes, leafy greens, and limes, if desired.

Homemade Taco Shells

Place a skillet over medium-high heat and add 1 tablespoon butter. Once the oil is heated, hold 1 tortilla with a pair of tongs and place half of it in the skillet. Hold it in a taco shape. Cook until it is golden brown. Repeat with the other side. When cooked, place over paper towels like a tent to drain.

Juicy Bison Burgers

Bison is one of the greatest meats of all time. With a perfect ratio of fat and protein, it's a meat that is incredible for nearly any application.

INGREDIENTS | SERVES 4

2 tablespoons butter, divided
½ cup shredded onion
¾ cup gluten-free bread crumbs
1 teaspoon coconut aminos
1 teaspoon Worcestershire sauce
½ teaspoon garlic powder
¼ teaspoon ground mustard
¼ teaspoon ground black pepper
1 teaspoon salt
¼ cup shredded zucchini
¼ cup mushrooms, minced
1 pound ground bison

1. Place a skillet over medium heat. Once it is heated, add 1 tablespoon butter and the onion. Cook for 5 minutes, or until very soft. Remove the skillet from the heat, and place the onion in a large bowl. Combine all other ingredients, except for the bison and other teaspoon of butter, and stir until well combined.

2. Break the bison over the surface of the bowl. Use your hands to gently massage the meat into the other ingredients. Combine the meat into four equally shaped balls.

3. Flatten balls into patties and then wrap them in plastic wrap. Place in the refrigerator to rest for at least 20 minutes.

4. Place a large cast-iron skillet over medium heat and add 1 tablespoon butter. Place patties into the skillet and cook for 4–5 minutes, or until well browned.

5. Flip patties, cover the skillet with a lid, and let cook for an additional 4–5 minutes. Check the center to make sure they are cooked to your liking.

Braised and Pan-Seared Duck Legs

This dish is more commonly known as duck confit, but only if you plan on keeping the meat in the jar with the fat in your refrigerator.

INGREDIENTS | SERVES 2

2 duck legs with skin on

¼ teaspoon salt

¼ teaspoon ground black pepper to taste

2 bay leaves, crumbled

Thumb-sized bundle of fresh thyme

Skin from remainder of duck

The Glory of Duck Fat

Duck fat rivals bacon fat for flavor but its higher smoke point makes it perfect for frying. Duck fat can be substituted in any vegetable recipe that requires 1–3 tablespoons of oil. Potatoes cooked in duck fat are the most flavorful you'll come across. They're perfect when served alongside steamed mussels and other French favorites.

1. Sprinkle the duck legs with salt and pepper. Place in an airtight container with bay leaves and thyme and refrigerate for 12–24 hours.

2. Place a skillet over medium-low heat. Once it is heated, add the skin to the skillet and cook for 1 hour, stirring occasionally to keep the fat from sticking. Cool for 15 minutes.

3. Preheat the oven to 300°F. Carefully place the duck legs in the skillet with the bay leaves and thyme. Place in the middle of the oven and cook for 2 hours, or until the bone moves independently of the meat.

4. Remove the pan from the oven and set it aside to cool. Pour off the fat.

5. Duck fat will keep for up to 2 months in an airtight container in the refrigerator.

Berry Spinach Salad

The flavor of fresh dill and fresh raspberries mingled together is quite an adventure for your taste buds! This salad spells summer and is great served for a special summer luncheon or supper. You can serve it as a side salad or an entrée.

INGREDIENTS | SERVES 6

6 cups fresh spinach
1 teaspoon toasted sesame seeds
2 cups fresh raspberries
¼ cup olive oil
2 tablespoons red wine vinegar
1½ teaspoons minced fresh dill
⅛ teaspoon onion powder
⅛ teaspoon garlic powder
⅛ teaspoon dry mustard
⅛ teaspoon salt (optional)

Razzy Raspberries

Raspberries have incredible nutritional value. They are a rich source of vitamin C and manganese. Most importantly, they are a low glycemic fruit that does not spike your blood sugar and cause a crash.

1. Wash the spinach carefully. Remove stems and heavy veins. Tear into bite-sized pieces.

2. Place spinach in a large bowl. Sprinkle with the toasted sesame seeds.

3. Add raspberries to the spinach.

4. In a screw top jar, combine the remaining ingredients. Shake until well mixed. Chill.

5. Shake dressing again and pour over spinach mixture. Toss gently. Garnish with a whole strawberry, if desired.

Papaya Salad

This is a very refreshing salad—not to mention a very pretty presentation—served in a scooped out papaya!

INGREDIENTS | SERVES 4

1 large papaya, diced into ½" cubes

1 small red bell pepper, chopped

2 medium stalks celery, diced

2 scallions, thinly sliced

1 pound fresh crab meat

1 cup plain yogurt

2 tablespoons honey

2 teaspoons orange zest

1 teaspoon cinnamon

1 orange, peeled and sectioned

1 kiwi fruit, peeled and sliced

1. In a bowl, combine the papaya, red pepper, celery, scallions, and crab meat. Place in refrigerator while making dressing.

2. In a small bowl, combine the yogurt, honey, orange zest, and cinnamon. Stir well to blend ingredients. Set aside.

3. Fill the papaya shells and garnish with the orange sections and sliced kiwi. Top with honey dressing. Chill before serving.

Papaya Trivia

This yellow-orange fruit contains papain, which is an enzyme similar to pepsin, the digestive juice. The seeds of papayas are usually thrown away; however, they can be dried and used like peppercorns. Papaya is very high in vitamin C and beta carotene.

Fresh Greens and Red Pepper Dressing

Take a little extra time to roast the red peppers—you won't be sorry!
If you do it once, you'll do it for many other recipes.

INGREDIENTS | SERVES 6

1 large red bell pepper
3 tablespoons white wine vinegar
2 tablespoons water
2 teaspoons olive oil
¼ teaspoon salt
⅛ teaspoon ground red pepper
1 tablespoon minced fresh basil
2 cups torn red leaf lettuce
2 cups torn green leaf lettuce
2 cups torn romaine lettuce
1 cup chopped tomato
1 cup chopped cucumber

1. Preheat oven to 425°F. Cut bell pepper in half lengthwise. Remove seeds and membrane. Place pepper, skin side up, on a foil-lined baking sheet. Bake for about 20 minutes or until skin is browned.

2. Cover with aluminum foil. Set aside and allow to cool. When bell pepper is cooled to room temperature, peel and discard skin.

3. Blend roasted pepper, vinegar, water, olive oil, salt, and red pepper until smooth. Place roasted pepper mixture in a small bowl. Stir in basil. Cover tightly and refrigerate for at least 60 minutes.

4. In a large bowl, combine lettuces, tomato, and cucumber. Toss gently.

5. Drizzle red pepper mixture over salad and serve immediately.

Smoked Turkey with Rosemary-Apple Salsa

The texture and flavor of a smoked wild bird are superb. Serve this with Rosemary-Apple Salsa or slice the meat and serve as a salad topper with all the fixings.

INGREDIENTS | SERVES 8

Salsa

1 large Granny Smith apple, cored and chopped

1 large tart red apple, cored and chopped

1 large yellow bell pepper, seeded and chopped

10 scallions, chopped

⅓ cup dried apricots, chopped

2 teaspoons fresh rosemary, finely chopped

¼ cup lemon juice

½ cup olive oil

½ teaspoon kosher salt

½ teaspoon freshly ground black pepper

Smoked Turkey

½ cup balsamic vinegar

2 tablespoons water

1 tablespoon paprika

1 tablespoon kosher salt

1 tablespoon lemon pepper

¼ teaspoon marjoram

4 pounds wild turkey breast halves, legs, and/or thighs

1. For the salsa: Combine all of the salsa ingredients in a large bowl. Toss to mix well. Cover with plastic wrap and refrigerate for 1–2 hours.

2. For the turkey: Combine the vinegar, water, paprika, salt, pepper, and marjoram in a glass jar and shake to blend.

3. Place the turkey pieces in a large resealable plastic bag. Pour the marinade into the bag and carefully seal the bag, removing most of the air. Refrigerate for 1–2 hours.

4. Build an indirect fire in a kettle grill or water smoker and add 3–4 water-soaked applewood chunks to the fire.

5. Remove the turkey pieces from the marinade and place on the indirect-heat side of the grill or smoker. Slow smoke at 225°F for about 1½–2 hours or until a thermometer inserted into the thickest portion of the breast meat and the thigh or leg meat registers 165°F–170°F for well-done.

6. The turkey will have a slightly pink color from the slow smoking and the wood. Slice and serve.

Leek, Mushroom, and Goat Cheese Quesadilla

The 6" cast-iron skillets fit a small corn tortilla perfectly. This one-pot lunch is a great quick meal for one and is easily adaptable.

INGREDIENTS | SERVES 1

2 tablespoons butter, divided
¼ cup leek, chopped
¼ cup mushrooms, chopped
½ teaspoon garlic powder
¼ teaspoon salt
¼ teaspoon ground black pepper
2 organic corn or rice flour tortillas
¼ cup goat cheese, crumbled
½ cup wheat-free salsa, optional

1. Place a small skillet over medium heat. Once heated add 1 tablespoon butter and leek. Cook for 3–4 minutes or until the leek is just starting to soften. Add the mushrooms, garlic powder, salt, and pepper and stir frequently for 4–5 minutes. The mushrooms should reduce and the leeks should start to turn golden.

2. Remove the contents of the skillet to a small bowl. Wipe out the skillet and add 1 tablespoon butter. Place 1 corn tortilla in the skillet and add the leek and mushroom mixture on top of it. Add the cheese on top, being careful to keep it from touching the sides of the skillet. Place another tortilla on top and press down.

3. Cook for 3–4 minutes, or until the bottom tortilla is crispy. Carefully remove the quesadilla from the skillet and flip over. Cook the second side for 2–3 minutes or until crispy.

4. Remove from skillet and let it rest for 3 minutes before slicing in half and serving with or without salsa.

Fish Drowned in Lemon Basil

There are many types of basil. Lemon basil has a delicate lemony flavor and can be hard to find. But any type of basil, other than Thai basil, can be substituted in this recipe.

INGREDIENTS | SERVES 4

4 (6-ounce) wild-caught tilapia fillets (or a similar white fish)

¼ teaspoon salt

¼ teaspoon ground black pepper

2–3 tablespoons butter

2 small zucchini or yellow squash, sliced

1 cup lemon basil leaves

Zest from 1 lemon

Juice from 1 lemon

Which Fish Is Best?

For people who rarely eat fish at home, shopping for fish can be overwhelming. But it shouldn't be. Fish is often served as either a steak (a cross-section of the gutted fish) or a fillet (meat from one half of a fish). White fish tends to have a less fishy taste on its own and picks up flavors from sauces very well.

1. Rinse the fish fillets and pat dry with paper towels. Squeeze gently to find any remaining bones and remove. Sprinkle lightly with salt and pepper. Set aside.

2. Place a large skillet over medium heat and add 2 tablespoons butter. Slide 2 fillets into the skillet and cook on each side for 4–5 minutes, or until the center is almost opaque and the fish begins to flake on the tips. Place on a clean plate to keep warm. Cook the remaining fish and add to the plate.

3. If all of the butter is gone from the skillet, add another tablespoon of butter to the pan before adding the zucchini rounds.

4. Sprinkle the basil, lemon zest, and a pinch of salt and pepper over the zucchini. Cover the pan and steam for 1 minute before tossing. Place the fish on top of the zucchini and sprinkle with lemon juice. Cover the skillet for 2–3 minutes to warm the fish and finish cooking the zucchini. Serve immediately.

Restaurant-Style Ribeye

This technique works well with almost any cut of tender steak. In addition to ribeye, you can use a New York strip, T-bone, porterhouse, tenderloin, or a filet mignon.

INGREDIENTS | SERVES 2

2 (1"-thick) choice-grade ribeye steaks
2 tablespoons butter, divided
¼ teaspoon salt
¼ teaspoon ground black pepper

Steak Temperatures

When following this recipe, begin testing the steak after cooking 3 minutes. Remove the steak when the center of the steak is done to these temperatures: rare: 120°F; medium-rare: 125°F; medium: 130°F; medium-well: 145°F; well: 155°F. The steak temperature will rise 5° while it rests.

1. Let your steaks sit at room temperature for 30 minutes before cooking. Preheat oven to 425°F. Place a cast-iron skillet large enough to hold two steaks on a burner over high heat. Turn on a vent if you have one or open a window.

2. Pat the steaks dry and brush both sides of each steak with 1 tablespoon butter. Sprinkle salt and pepper on each side of the steaks. Test the skillet temperature by placing a drop of water in the center. If it sizzles, you know it's ready. Place the steaks in the skillet so they aren't touching and let them sit without moving for 2 minutes. Carefully flip each steak over. Cook on the other side for 2 minutes.

3. Turn off the burner. Cut remaining butter into two pieces and put a piece on the middle of each steak. Move the skillet to the middle of your oven. The cut, thickness, and quality of the meat will determine cooking time.

4. Once the steaks are done, place them on a plate, cover with a piece of foil, and let them rest for 5 minutes.

CHAPTER 12

Dinner

Mushroom Pork Medallions

You would never guess this meal is packed with superfoods. It tastes so amazing, you will swear it was deep fried with flour.

INGREDIENTS | SERVES 2

1 pound pork tenderloin
1 tablespoon olive oil
1 small onion, peeled and sliced
¼ cup sliced fresh mushrooms
1 clove garlic, minced
2 teaspoons flax meal
½ cup unsalted beef broth
¼ teaspoon dried rosemary, crushed
⅛ teaspoon ground black pepper

1. Slice tenderloin into ½" thick medallions.

2. In a skillet, heat olive oil over medium-high heat. Brown pork in oil 2 minutes on each side.

3. Remove pork from skillet and set aside.

4. In same skillet, add onion, mushrooms, and garlic and sauté 1 minute.

5. Stir in flax meal until blended.

6. Gradually stir in the broth, rosemary, and pepper. Bring to a boil; cook and stir 1 minute or until thickened.

7. Lay pork medallions over mixture. Reduce heat; cover and simmer 15 minutes or until meat juices run clear.

Grass-Fed Lamb Meatballs

Meatballs are always a kid favorite. These grass-fed lamb meatballs are high in good fats that contribute to their taste and their health factor.

INGREDIENTS | SERVES 6

¼ cup pine nuts
4 tablespoons olive oil, divided
1½ pounds ground grass-fed lamb
¼ cup minced garlic
2 tablespoons cumin

1. Over medium-high heat sauté pine nuts in 2 tablespoons olive oil 2 minutes until brown. Remove from pan and allow to cool.

2. In a large bowl, combine lamb, garlic, cumin, and pine nuts and form into meatballs.

3. Add remaining olive oil to pan and fry meatballs until cooked through, about 5–10 minutes, depending on size of meatballs.

Spicy Grilled Flank Steak

Flank steak is one of the leanest steak cuts. It is usually the best and safest choice of steak to order when going out to dinner, as well.

INGREDIENTS | SERVES 4

2 tablespoons raw honey
1 teaspoon cinnamon
1 teaspoon chili powder
½ teaspoon salt-free lemon pepper seasoning
1½ pounds lean flank steak
½ cup sliced green onions

1. Combine honey, cinnamon, chili powder, and lemon pepper seasoning in a small bowl.

2. Grill flank steak over medium-high heat covered for 6 minutes on each side. Baste often with honey mixture.

3. Serve sprinkled with green onions as garnish.

Flank Steak and Good Fat

Flank steak is a terrific choice when you want a lower-fat version of red meat. This steak usually contains less than 13 grams of fat per serving, while some other more fatty cuts have about 20 grams of fat per serving.

Shrimp Skewers

These skewers are easy to make and can be served as a main dish or an appetizer. They are fantastic at parties or holiday celebrations.

INGREDIENTS | SERVES 4

1½ pounds large shrimp, peeled and deveined

Juice of ½ lime

1 teaspoon ground black pepper

1 medium zucchini, sliced in 1" pieces

1 medium summer squash, sliced in 1" pieces

1 large red bell pepper, sliced in 2" × 2" pieces

1 large green bell pepper, sliced in 2" × 2" pieces

4 cloves garlic, peeled and finely minced

2 tablespoons olive oil

1. Soak 8 wooden skewers in water for at least 30 minutes.

2. In a large bowl, drizzle shrimp with lime juice and season with black pepper. Set aside for 5 minutes.

3. Add vegetables, garlic, and olive oil to the shrimp and toss to coat.

4. Alternate vegetables and shrimp on skewers.

5. Grill over medium heat 5 minutes or until shrimp turns pink, then turn skewers to cook other side an additional 5 minutes.

Shrimp and Omega-3

Shrimp is a good source of omega-3 fatty acids. This terrific shellfish is naturally low in fat and high in protein. If you have high cholesterol, you might want to watch your intake. They do have higher levels than other protein sources.

Barbecue Chicken

This mouthwatering chicken will become a staple in your home regardless of the season.

INGREDIENTS | SERVES 4

3 tablespoons olive oil
1½ cups apple cider vinegar
½ cup raw honey
Juice of 1 medium lemon
¼ teaspoon ground black pepper
5 fresh sage sprigs
2 pounds bone-in chicken breasts

1. In a small bowl combine olive oil, vinegar, honey, lemon juice, pepper, and sage.

2. Place chicken breasts on hot grill and baste with sauce.

3. Cook for 45–60 minutes, turning every 10–15 minutes. Baste with sauce after each turning.

Cage-Free and Barn-Roaming

Cage-free and barn-roaming chickens are the best chickens to purchase. Chickens that are given feedlot grains derived from corn have a less attractive fat profile. Commercial farms tend to use antibiotics and growth hormones. All of these products eventually leach into our bodies where they can magnify over time.

Pulled Chicken

This chicken will melt in your mouth after hours in the slow cooker.

INGREDIENTS | SERVES 8

2 pounds barn-roaming chicken breast
1 (16-ounce) can diced tomatoes
1 cup diced sweet onion
4 carrots, cut into large pieces
2 green onions
4 cloves garlic, peeled and cut coarsely
1 tablespoon thyme
1 teaspoon chili powder

1. Combine all ingredients into slow cooker and cook on high 5 hours.

2. Shred chicken with forks before serving, and toss to coat in the vegetable mixture.

3. Reduce heat and serve.

Rosemary Rack of Lamb in Berries Sauce

This rack of lamb recipe is sure to be a winner at any holiday or dinner party. The flavors are strong and the presentation a winner.

INGREDIENTS | SERVES 4

1 rack of grass-fed lamb, on the bone
¼ teaspoon fresh ground black pepper
2 cloves crushed garlic, divided
¼ teaspoon dried thyme
2 sprigs fresh rosemary
2 tablespoons olive oil
1 cup mixed berries of your choice
1 cup unsalted organic beef stock

1. Preheat oven to 400°F.

2. On the rack of lamb, sprinkle black pepper, 1 clove crushed garlic, thyme, and 1 sprig of fresh rosemary.

3. Place lamb in oven. Roast for 13 minutes per pound or until internal temperature reaches 135°F. Remove from oven and set aside to rest.

4. Prepare sauce by combining remaining garlic, rosemary, olive oil, berries, and beef stock in a medium pan over low heat. Stir and cook about 5 minutes.

5. Reduce sauce until thick (may take another 5 minutes) and pour over cooked lamb.

Curried Shrimp with Veggies

This curried shrimp and vegetable dish is quick and easy, but quite authentic-tasting. It is sure to please everyone in your family who is fond of foods from India.

INGREDIENTS | SERVES 4

2 tablespoons olive oil

1 tablespoon green curry powder

1 pound wild Argentinian shrimp, peeled and deveined

1 (12-ounce) bag frozen broccoli florets

4 large carrots, sliced

1 (8-ounce) can coconut milk

1. In a large skillet over medium heat, warm olive oil and green curry powder.

2. Add shrimp, broccoli, carrots, and coconut milk.

3. Cook until all vegetables are tender and coconut milk cooks down to a thick, paste-like consistency, approximately 15 minutes.

Steamed King Crab Legs

Shellfish is a healthy and flavorful protein source. It is naturally low in fat and has a nice, sweet taste—a great alternative to the usual poultry or beef dish.

INGREDIENTS | SERVES 4

2 tablespoons oil

3 cloves garlic, peeled and crushed

1 (1") piece fresh gingerroot, crushed

1 stalk lemongrass, crushed

2 pounds Alaskan king crab legs

1 teaspoon ground black pepper

1. Heat oil in a large pot over medium-high heat.

2. Add garlic, ginger, and lemongrass; cook and stir until brown, about 5 minutes.

3. Add crab legs and pepper. Cover and cook, tossing occasionally, for 15 minutes.

Spicy Chicken Burgers

You can substitute ground turkey or pork for the chicken. Adjust the quantity of pepper flakes to control the spiciness.

INGREDIENTS | SERVES 4

1 pound ground chicken breast
¼ cup finely chopped yellow onion
¼ cup finely chopped red bell pepper
1 teaspoon minced garlic
¼ cup thinly sliced scallions
½ teaspoon hot pepper flakes
¼ teaspoon freshly cracked black pepper

1. Clean and oil broiler rack. Preheat broiler to medium.

2. Combine all ingredients in a medium-sized bowl, mixing lightly. Broil the burgers for 4–5 minutes per side until firm through the center and the juices run clear. Transfer to a plate and tent with foil to keep warm. Allow to rest 1–2 minutes before serving.

Chicken Stew with Meat Sauce

This easy-to-make chicken stew is sure to please the entire family. Both kids and adults love this delicious recipe. Serve alone or pour over spaghetti squash as a bolognese-type sauce.

INGREDIENTS | SERVES 4

1 pound (90% lean) grass-fed ground beef

4 boneless, skinless chicken breasts

1 (6-ounce) can organic tomato paste

1 (28-ounce) can diced organic tomatoes, no salt added

4 cloves garlic, peeled and minced

4 large carrots, sliced

2 medium red bell peppers, seeded and diced

2 medium green bell peppers, seeded and diced

1 tablespoon dried thyme

2 tablespoons olive oil

1 tablespoon chili powder

1. In a medium sauté pan over medium heat, cook ground beef until browned, about 5 minutes. Drain and place in slow cooker.

2. Wipe out pan and place over medium-high heat. Brown the chicken breasts, 5 minutes per side. Add to slow cooker.

3. Combine all remaining ingredients in slow cooker.

4. Cook on high 5 hours.

5. Serve over your favorite steamed vegetable.

Slow Cookers Are Lifesavers

A slow cooker is a great appliance for a busy lifestyle. These little countertop cookers allow you to cook easily and in bulk, which can be handy when planning meals for hectic schedules.

Red Rice and Sausage

This recipe is so easy—and perfect for when you are low on time. Kids love it and grown-ups do too.

INGREDIENTS | SERVES 4–6

1 pound sweet or hot Italian sausage, cut into 1" pieces

1 medium onion, peeled and finely chopped

2 cloves garlic, peeled and chopped

Small amount olive oil (optional)

1 cup red rice, uncooked

2¾ cups chicken broth

1 teaspoon dried rosemary or 1 tablespoon fresh rosemary

½ cup grated Parmesan cheese

¼ cup chopped fresh parsley

1. Brown sausage pieces, onion, and garlic in oven-safe skillet over medium-high heat for 5–8 minutes. If sausage is very lean, add a bit of olive oil to prevent the food from sticking.

2. Stir in rice and toss with sausage and vegetables. Add broth and rosemary and cover. Cook on very low heat or place in a 325°F oven for 45–60 minutes.

3. Just before serving, sprinkle the top with Parmesan cheese and brown under the broiler. Add chopped parsley and serve.

What Is Red Rice?

Yes, there is more out there than white or brown rice! Red rice is often found in Europe, Southeast Asia, and India. Red rice has a similar nutritional profile as brown rice, as they are both high in fiber. When red rice is cooked, the natural red color of the bran leeches out and turns the rest of the rice a reddish-pink color.

Ginger, Soy, and Kale Chicken

This recipe has a wonderful combination of ginger and soy. Marinate it the night before to let the chicken thoroughly absorb the flavors.

INGREDIENTS | SERVES 2

4 tablespoons low-sodium wheat-free soy sauce

1 tablespoon toasted sesame oil

1 tablespoon honey

½ teaspoon fresh grated gingerroot

2 cloves garlic, peeled and crushed

2 boneless, skinless organic chicken breasts, cut into 1" cubes

1 tablespoon extra-virgin olive oil

2 cups kale

Are You Familiar with Kale?

Kale is a powerhouse of nutrition as well as being a member of the cabbage family. Kale is packed with fiber, calcium, vitamin B_6, vitamin A, vitamin K, and vitamin C. Kale can be eaten raw or cooked and can replace your other leafy greens in all varieties of recipes.

1. In a small bowl, whisk together soy sauce, sesame oil, honey, gingerroot, and garlic.

2. Place chicken in a zip-top plastic bag and pour half of the soy mixture into bag. Make sure the bag is closed and shake it up so all the chicken is covered. Let marinate for at least a half hour or overnight.

3. Remove chicken from the marinade. Heat olive oil in a large skillet over medium-high heat. Sauté chicken for 5–8 minutes, until fully cooked and no longer pink.

4. Add kale and cook until it is still bright green but only a little soft, about 2 minutes. Add remaining soy mixture and mix well.

Hot and Spicy Turkey Meatballs

Meatball recipes usually include bread crumbs as a filler and sometimes for an outside coating. This recipe uses ground potato chips. The eggs will hold the meatballs together, and who doesn't love potato chips?

INGREDIENTS | MAKES 10–12 MEATBALLS

1 pound ground turkey

2 large eggs

2 cloves garlic, peeled and minced

1 teaspoon dried oregano

1 teaspoon dried basil

½ teaspoon cinnamon

½ teaspoon fennel seeds

½ cup finely grated raw Parmesan cheese

2 cups crushed low-salt potato chips, divided

½ teaspoon Himalayan salt

½ teaspoon ground black pepper

4 tablespoons butter

1. In a large bowl, mix turkey, eggs, garlic, oregano, basil, cinnamon, fennel seeds, cheese, 1 cup potato chip crumbs, salt, and pepper.

2. Place a large sheet of waxed paper on the counter. Sprinkle remaining cup of chip crumbs on it.

3. Form 1" meatballs from the turkey mixture. Roll meatballs in crumbs to coat.

4. Heat butter in a large skillet over medium-high heat. Fry meatballs until well browned, about 5 minutes. Drain on paper towels and then either refrigerate, freeze, or serve with the marinara sauce of your choice.

Kick Up Those Meatballs

You can add flavor to your meatballs by grinding up some sweet or hot Italian sausage and mixing it with the ground turkey or beef. A truly great Italian sausage has aromatics like garlic and herbs, and spices such as anise seeds.

Garlic Balsamic Crusted Pork Tenderloin

This is wonderful for entertaining. Mashed potatoes and roasted vegetables pair perfectly with this tenderloin.

INGREDIENTS | SERVES 4

3 cloves garlic, peeled and minced

2 tablespoons balsamic vinegar

½ teaspoon ground mustard powder

1 teaspoon Himalayan salt

¼ teaspoon ground black pepper

2 tablespoons extra-virgin olive oil, divided

1–1¼ pounds pork tenderloin

2 tablespoons fresh parsley, for garnish (optional)

1. In a small bowl, mix together garlic, balsamic vinegar, mustard, salt, pepper and 1 tablespoon olive oil. Rub the paste all over pork. Marinate for at least 2–3 hours or overnight if you'd like.

2. Preheat oven to 400°F. Heat remaining oil in large skillet over medium-high heat. Working in batches if necessary, add pork and brown tenderloin all over, about 4–5 minutes.

3. Transfer pan to preheated oven. Roast pork, turning occasionally, until the internal temperature reaches 160°F, about 20–30 minutes.

4. Transfer pork to a cutting board and let rest 10 minutes before slicing. Top with fresh parsley if desired.

Ginger-Teriyaki Flank Steak

This Asian-inspired dish pairs perfectly with steamed vegetables and rice. This marinade can be used on a variety of meats such as chicken, pork, and other cuts of beef.

INGREDIENTS | SERVES 4

½ cup water

1 tablespoon sesame oil

½ teaspoon grated gingerroot

2 cloves garlic, peeled and minced

¼ cup wheat-free soy sauce

1 tablespoon honey

1 tablespoon cornstarch

1½ pounds beef flank steak

What Does It Mean to Slice Against the Grain?

Lines in the flank steak run from right to left down the length of the steak. By cutting across these lines, the knife will cut through the fibers, which makes it easier to chew. Slicing the steak on a 45°-angle creates an elegant presentation.

1. In a small bowl, mix water, sesame oil, gingerroot, garlic, soy sauce, honey, and cornstarch. Stir thoroughly to ensure the cornstarch has been mixed in well.

2. Place the steak in zip-top bag and pour the marinade on top. Make sure the bag is sealed and shake until well blended. Place in refrigerator and let sit for at least 4 hours or, even better, overnight.

3. When ready to cook the steaks, remove them from the bag and discard the leftover marinade.

4. Place steaks on preheated grill or on a grill pan and cook on each side for about 6–8 minutes, until you have reached your desired degree of doneness. The internal temperature should read at least 145°F.

Spicy Steak Fajitas

Skirt steak rubbed with spicy seasoning and chopped peppers and served with warmed corn tortillas makes for the perfect family meal.

INGREDIENTS | SERVES 8

1 tablespoon cornstarch
2 teaspoons chili powder
1 teaspoon salt
1 teaspoon paprika
½ teaspoon red pepper flakes
1 teaspoon wheat-free Worcestershire sauce
1 teaspoon fresh lime juice
1 teaspoon turbinado sugar
¼ teaspoon cumin
3 pounds skirt steak
4 cloves garlic, peeled and minced
½ medium onion, peeled and chopped
1 medium green bell pepper, sliced
1 medium red or yellow bell pepper, sliced
½ bunch fresh cilantro
Corn tortillas
10 ounces shredded raw Monterey jack cheese

1. In a small bowl, mix cornstarch, chili powder, salt, paprika, red pepper flakes, Worcestershire sauce, lime juice, sugar, and cumin.

2. Rub steaks with garlic and the prepared seasoning mixture then cut it into strips.

3. Heat oil in a large skillet over medium heat. Cook onion, peppers, and cilantro for 3–4 minutes. Add steak strips and cook, stirring frequently, until cooked through, about 7 minutes.

4. Remove from heat and spoon meat into a corn tortilla. Top with cheese and roll up.

Slow Cooker Pulled Pork

You will love how your house smells when this is slow cooking.
Feel free to use chicken if you don't eat pork.

INGREDIENTS | SERVES 6

2 medium yellow onions, peeled and chopped

5 cloves garlic, peeled and minced

1 cup beef broth

1 tablespoon brown sugar

1 tablespoon chili powder

2 teaspoons kosher salt

1 teaspoon cumin

½ teaspoon cinnamon

½ teaspoon dried oregano

1 (5-pound) pork shoulder, boneless or bone-in

1 cup wheat-free barbecue sauce

1 teaspoon wheat-free soy sauce

Wheat-free buns or tortillas

1. Place onions, garlic, and broth in a slow cooker.

2. In a small bowl, combine the sugar, chili powder, salt, cumin, cinnamon, and oregano and mix well.

3. Pat pork with a paper towel and rub prepared mixture all over it. Place pork on top of broth in slow cooker.

4. In the same small bowl, mix the barbecue sauce and the soy sauce. Stir to combine. Pour on top of pork making sure the mixture is spread evenly on top. Cover and cook on low 8 hours.

5. Remove pork from slow cooker and allow to cool slightly. If using bone-in pork, discard bone. Place pork in 9" × 13" casserole dish.

6. Shred the pork using a fork. Add additional barbecue sauce and slow cooker mixture if you'd like. Serve warm in wheat-free buns or tortillas.

Baby Back Ribs

You can use any kind of barbecue sauce you wish for this recipe. The trick is to cook the ribs in the sauce.

INGREDIENTS | SERVES 4–6

4 pounds baby back ribs, cut into 1-rib servings

½ cup coconut oil

1 cup Easy Barbecue Sauce (see recipe in this chapter)

1 teaspoon garlic powder

1 cup tomato juice

1. Fry ribs in coconut oil over medium-high heat until lightly brown, about 3–4 minutes each side.

2. Add rest of ingredients and cover. Cook over very low heat for 1 hour.

3. Remove ribs and continue cooking the sauce until reduced to 1 cup, about 5–8 minutes. Serve sauce with ribs for dipping.

Easy Barbecue Sauce

You will never want store-bought barbecue sauce again after you make this. This zesty sauce is perfect for chicken, pork, or beef. You can keep this in an airtight container in the refrigerator for a few weeks.

INGREDIENTS | MAKES 8 SERVINGS (1 CUP)

1 tablespoon cider vinegar

½ cup ketchup

1 tablespoon raw honey

2 tablespoons brown sugar

1 teaspoon garlic powder

½ tablespoon onion powder

1 tablespoon red pepper flakes

2 tablespoons wheat-free Worcestershire sauce

¼ teaspoon Himalayan salt

1. Place all ingredients in a small saucepan over medium heat.

2. Bring to a boil, turn heat to low, and simmer on low for a few minutes, stirring.

3. Allow to cool before brushing onto meat.

Grilled Chicken Wings

Traditional Buffalo wings are generally fried. This recipe, done with a rub and some olive oil, is a lot less fattening. Double the recipe and refrigerate half for delicious cold snacks.

INGREDIENTS | SERVES 4–8

4 pounds chicken wings, split at the joint, tips removed

1 tablespoon onion powder

1 tablespoon garlic powder

¼ teaspoon cinnamon

2 teaspoons dark brown sugar

½ teaspoon paprika

½ teaspoon ground black pepper

¼ cup freshly squeezed lime juice

¼ cup extra-virgin olive oil

1 teaspoon Himalayan salt

¼ teaspoon ground black pepper

1. Rinse wings and set them on paper towels to dry.

2. In a large bowl, mix rest of ingredients together. Coat chicken with spice mixture, cover, and refrigerate 1 hour.

3. Grill over medium-hot coals or broil at 350°F 20 minutes, turning every few minutes, or until well browned.

Olive Oil in Spray Bottles

This is a very easy and economical way to use olive oil. Just buy a bottle used for spraying plants with water and fill it with olive oil instead. Use it for spraying your food, salads, and so on. Or you can get olive oil–flavored nonstick spray at the supermarket. The nonstick spray, however, is not suitable for salads.

Peppered Buffalo Tenderloin

A large animal has a large tenderloin. This makes a lot and is great for a crowd. But the leftovers are wonderful to make a salad or sandwich for noshing on the weekend.

INGREDIENTS | SERVES 12–14

2 tablespoons coarse kosher salt

6 tablespoons cracked black pepper

1 (8-pound) buffalo tenderloin

9 tablespoons unsalted butter

3 tablespoons olive oil

1 cup brandy

Buffalo

Though wild until it was near extinction in the late 1800s, there are some free-ranging herds in protected parks. The buffalo that graces your table is domestically raised. The animals are hardy and are usually not given any hormones or antibiotics. The meat has half the cholesterol of beef.

1. Evenly press salt and pepper all over tenderloin.

2. In a large (flat surface) roasting pan heat butter and oil and sauté the tenderloin over high to medium-high heat. Cook about 20–30 minutes, searing on all sides until cooked rare or medium-rare.

3. Place tenderloin on a cutting board to rest. Heat juices in roasting pan and add brandy. Bring to a boil and simmer over medium heat for 5 minutes.

4. Slice tenderloin in ½"-thick slices. Arrange on a platter and pour warm pan juices over all.

Skillet Burgers with Tarragon Butter

Serve burgers on good-quality gluten-free kaiser rolls, focaccia, ciabatta, or crusty bakery rolls. Don't forget to shape the burgers to fit the buns.

INGREDIENTS | SERVES 6

½ cup (1 stick) unsalted butter, softened

2 green onions, chopped

2 tablespoons chopped parsley

2 teaspoons chopped fresh tarragon

2 teaspoons tarragon vinegar

¼ teaspoon seasoned pepper

6 gluten-free hamburger buns

1½ pounds ground big-game meat like buffalo or venison

Kosher salt and pepper

Tomato slices, red onion slices, and chopped lettuce, to top burgers

1. Combine butter, onions, parsley, fresh tarragon, tarragon vinegar, and seasoned pepper to taste. Butter the hamburger buns and set aside.

2. Form ground meat into 6 patties to fit hamburger buns. Salt and pepper both sides of each burger.

3. Heat a heavy-duty skillet over high heat. Place burgers in skillet and sear over high heat for about 3 minutes per side for rare, 4 minutes per side for medium, and 5–6 minutes per side for well-done.

4. While the burgers are cooking, broil or toast the hamburger buns. Serve burgers on buns with the toppings of your choice.

Vinegar and Salt Brined Rotisserie Tenderloin

Invite a crowd over for this delicious meat that is slow cooked on a motorized spit. Figure ½ pound meat per person.

INGREDIENTS | SERVES A CROWD

1 tenderloin of wild big game like venison, antelope, or moose

1 quart Vinegar and Salt Brine (see sidebar)

½ cup (1 stick) butter, melted

2 cloves garlic, peeled and minced

1 tablespoon soy sauce

Vinegar and Salt Brine

Combine 1 quart water; 3 cups cider vinegar; ½ cup kosher salt; ⅓ cup dark brown sugar; 1 tablespoon black peppercorns; 1 bunch Italian parsley, chopped; 1 onion, chopped; 2 carrots, chopped; and 2 stalks celery, chopped, in a pot and bring to a boil. Turn off heat and let cool. Strain liquid and discard vegetables. Brine the big game of your choice for 12 hours to 2 or 3 days in the brining liquid in the refrigerator.

1. Place tenderloin in brine mixture and refrigerate 10–15 hours. Remove from marinade, rinse well, and pat dry.

2. Follow manufacturer's rotisserie directions: Secure clamp and fork at one end of rotisserie rod; slide rod through center of meat. Attach the other fork and secure clamp. Make sure meat is balanced. Tie up loose pieces of meat with string. Rotisserie cook at 350°F over a pan of water with the lid closed.

3. Combine melted butter, garlic, and soy sauce. Baste tenderloin every 15 minutes. Cook until rare or medium-rare as identified with a meat thermometer for best juiciness and tenderness. Let meat rest 15 minutes, then slice and serve. (Variation: Tenderloin may be grilled directly over the fire, turning every 5–7 minutes to sear all over until desired doneness.)

Grilled Venison Chops or Steaks with Butter

Have game steaks cut about ½" to ¾" thick. They will cook quickly and be less chewy.

INGREDIENTS | SERVES 4

2 tablespoons olive oil

4 venison chops or steaks, or other big game

2 tablespoons Coarse Kosher Salt and Freshly Cracked Pepper Rub (see sidebar)

1 tablespoon butter, divided

Coarse Kosher Salt and Freshly Cracked Pepper Rub

Combine ¼ cup coarse kosher salt, 2 tablespoons freshly cracked black peppercorns, and 2 tablespoons freshly cracked green peppercorns in a glass jar with a tight-fitting lid. Shake to blend. Will keep for several months.

1. Prepare a hot fire in the grill.

2. Rub olive oil on meat and sprinkle with salt and pepper rub. Set aside.

3. Grill meat for about 3–4 minutes per side for rare to medium-rare. Serve with a ¼ tablespoon of butter on top of each chop or steak.

Salt and Pepper Venison Steaks

Simplicity lets the flavor of the food shine. Try this recipe with the meat pan sautéed or seared over a hot charcoal fire.

INGREDIENTS | SERVES 4

8 deer tenderloin steaks, ½" thick

¼ teaspoon coarse kosher salt

¼ teaspoon freshly cracked black pepper

2 tablespoons olive oil

2 tablespoons unsalted butter

1. Season steaks with salt and pepper.

2. Heat oil and butter in a heavy skillet over medium-high heat. Place 4 steaks in the hot skillet at a time. Sear for about 2 minutes per side, turning only once. Repeat and cook remaining steaks. Serve hot.

Internal Meat Temperatures

Use a meat thermometer to ensure perfectly cooked meat. Most meat and game have less fat than domesticated animals do. Lean tender cuts become dry and tough if overcooked. Cook tenderloins for about 12–15 minutes per pound. Most game hunters and eaters prefer rare to medium-rare for optimum tenderness and juiciness: 125°F for rare, 130°F–140°F for medium-rare, 145°F–155°F for medium, and 160°F for well-done.

Rocky Mountain Hunter's Stew

Hunter's stew was typically made with a hodgepodge of leftover game meat. So if your refrigerator or freezer has any leftover cooked game, add it to the pot. To heighten and brighten the flavor of soups and stews, add some lemon zest and juice.

INGREDIENTS | SERVES 10–12

3 pounds stew meat, a combination of big-game meat

8 tablespoons butter, divided

1 pound game sausage or Italian sausage, sliced into 1" pieces

2 medium onions, peeled and chopped

8 ounces porcini mushrooms, sliced

3 carrots, peeled and finely chopped

1 (28-ounce) can fire-roasted tomatoes, chopped

4 (10-ounce) cans chicken stock

¼ teaspoon coarse kosher salt

¼ teaspoon freshly cracked black pepper

1. Trim excess fat off stew meat. In a medium sauté pan over medium high heat, sauté in melted butter in two batches to sear and lightly brown, 3–5 minutes. Set stew meat aside. Add game sausage and heat through. Set aside.

2. Add 4 more tablespoons butter to pot. Sauté onions and mushrooms for 3–4 minutes. Add rest of ingredients and bring to a boil. Reduce heat to low, cover, and simmer for 1½–2 hours, stirring occasionally. If stew is too thick, add 1–2 cups of water to thin down.

Rocky Mountains

The soaring range known as the Rocky Mountains stretches from western Canada into New Mexico. It is abundant with wildlife, especially big game. The conservation folks do a splendid job overseeing the management of the wild game, which includes keeping the game numbers in control and the animals safe from disease.

CHAPTER 13

Snacks and Sides

Party Guacamole

Guacamole is a party favorite that is quite healthy. Try serving with sliced bell peppers for dipping, or alongside your favorite fajita recipe.

INGREDIENTS | SERVES 4–6

4 ripe avocados
2 medium vine-ripe tomatoes, diced
½ cup diced green onions
1 tablespoon diced jalapeño peppers
2 cloves garlic, peeled and diced
Juice of 1 medium lime
¼ teaspoon ground black pepper

1. Scoop out avocado flesh and place in a small bowl. Mash the avocado with a fork.

2. Add tomatoes, onions, jalapeños, and garlic. Mix together.

3. Squeeze on fresh lime juice and mix.

4. Add black pepper and serve.

Antioxidant Fruit and Nut Salad

Fruit salad can be eaten any time of day, but is particularly good for breakfast. Berries are packed full of antioxidants and walnuts have one of the best omega profiles for nuts to reduce inflammation. This is a winning combination.

INGREDIENTS | SERVES 2

½ cup sliced strawberries
½ cup raspberries
½ cup blackberries
½ cup blueberries
½ cup dried mulberries
½ cup chopped walnuts

Combine all ingredients and enjoy.

Cacao Nib Cookies

If you are looking for a sweet treat try these Paleo cookies. These can be taken anywhere on the go and will give you satisfaction for your sweet tooth cravings.

INGREDIENTS | YIELDS 24 COOKIES

1 cup almond butter
⅔ cup shredded coconut
1½ tablespoons coconut oil
½ cup almond butter
1 cup cacao nibs
⅓ cup coconut flour
½ teaspoon cinnamon
1 large egg
2 tablespoons cacao powder
½ cup raw honey

1. Preheat oven to 350°F. Spray a cookie sheet with nonstick cooking spray.

2. Combine all ingredients into a large mixing bowl.

3. Spoon rounded teaspoon-sized balls onto prepared cookie sheet.

4. Cook 9 minutes. Cool before serving.

Coconut Cacao Cookies

When you're craving a sweet chocolate treat, try these coconut cacao cookies. They are quick and satisfying.

INGREDIENTS | YIELDS 12–14 COOKIES

7 pitted dates
½ cup shredded, unsweetened coconut
¾ cup almond flour
¼ cup coconut flour
1 teaspoon coconut oil
2 tablespoons coconut milk
1 large egg
1 cup cacao nibs

1. Preheat oven to 350°F.

2. Combine dates and unsweetened coconut in food processor and pulse until crumb-like consistency.

3. Pour mixture into a large mixing bowl and add remaining ingredients. Mix well with hands.

4. Form into patties and place on baking sheet sprayed with nonstick cooking spray.

5. Bake 22 minutes. Cool before serving.

Citrus-Steamed Carrots

Sweet figs and carrots are balanced with the tang of orange, lemon, and lime juice in this recipe.

INGREDIENTS | SERVES 6

1 cup orange juice
2 tablespoons lemon juice
2 tablespoons lime juice
1 pound carrots, peeled and julienned
3 fresh figs
1 tablespoon extra-virgin olive oil
1 tablespoon capers

1. In a medium pot, combine citrus juices and heat on medium-high. Add carrots, cover, and steam until al dente. Remove from heat and let cool.

2. Cut figs into wedges. Mound carrots on serving plates and arrange figs around carrots. Sprinkle olive oil and capers on top, and serve.

Baked Apples

You will feel as if you're eating apple pie when you eat these, and your house will smell like Thanksgiving dinner whenever you make them.

INGREDIENTS | SERVES 6

6 Pink Lady apples
1 cup unsweetened coconut flakes
¼ teaspoon ground cinnamon

1. Preheat oven to 350°F.

2. Remove cores to ½" of bottom of apples.

3. Place apples in a medium baking dish. Fill cores with coconut flakes and sprinkle with cinnamon.

4. Bake 10–15 minutes. Apples are done when they are completely soft and brown on top.

Broccoli, Pine Nut, and Apple Salad

This quick little salad will tide you over to your next meal. The broccoli and apple taste great together and the toasted pine nuts add a little bit of crunch.

INGREDIENTS | SERVES 2

4 tablespoons olive oil
¾ cup pine nuts
2 cups broccoli florets
2 cups diced green apples
Juice of 1 lemon

1. Heat olive oil in a small frying pan over medium heat and sauté pine nuts until golden brown.

2. Mix broccoli and apples in a medium bowl. Add pine nuts and toss.

3. Squeeze lemon juice over salad and serve.

Fresh Pepper Salsa

Tomatoes are a great source of the antioxidant vitamin C. You can also get creative and make your salsa with other vegetables, fruits, and spices.

INGREDIENTS | YIELDS 1 PINT

1 medium yellow bell pepper
1 medium orange bell pepper
1–2 poblano chilies
2 Anaheim chilies
1–2 jalapeño peppers
2 cloves garlic, peeled
¼ medium red onion
Juice of ½ medium lime
¼ teaspoon freshly crushed black pepper
Canola oil (enough to coat the pan)
1 tablespoon chopped cilantro

1. Place all ingredients (except oil and cilantro) in a food processor and pulse until desired chunkiness results. Taste and adjust for saltiness and heat.

2. In a medium pot, heat oil over medium-high heat until slightly smoking. Add blended pepper mixture. Cook on high 8–10 minutes, stirring occasionally. Sprinkle some chopped cilantro on top, if desired. Serve hot, cold, or at room temperature with tortilla chips, as a garnish for fish or poultry, or in your favorite burrito.

Trail Mix

For kids who love potato chips, this recipe will be a nice alternative. It has a sweet and salty taste to satisfy all their cravings.

INGREDIENTS | SERVES 8

½ cup cashews
½ cup almonds
½ cup macadamia nuts
½ cup pistachio nuts
4 tablespoons raw honey
1 teaspoon sea salt
½ teaspoon ground black pepper
¼ teaspoon ground cumin
1 teaspoon curry powder
⅛ teaspoon ground cloves
1 teaspoon ground cinnamon

1. Preheat oven to 300°F.

2. Place all nuts on a large baking sheet and bake 10–12 minutes, taking care they do not burn. Remove from oven and let cool approximately 5 minutes.

3. In a small bowl, mix honey, salt, pepper, cumin, curry powder, cloves, and cinnamon.

4. In a large saucepan over medium heat, place the nuts and half of the honey mixture. When the mixture begins to melt, mix in the remaining honey mixture.

5. Shake the pan until all the nuts are coated, about 5 minutes.

6. Cool on wax paper. Use a spoon to separate nuts that stick together.

Roasted Spicy Pumpkin Seeds

This spicy seed recipe is sure to be a favorite with the family for snacking.
They are quick to prepare and easy to grab for snacks on the go.

INGREDIENTS | SERVES 8

3 cups raw pumpkin seeds
½ cup olive oil
½ teaspoon garlic powder
¼ teaspoon ground black pepper

Pumpkin Seed Benefits

Pumpkin seeds have great health benefits. They contain L-Tryptophan, a compound found to naturally fight depression, and they are high in zinc, a mineral that protects against osteoporosis.

1. Preheat oven to 300°F.

2. In a medium bowl, mix together pumpkin seeds, olive oil, garlic powder, and black pepper until pumpkin seeds are evenly coated.

3. Spread in an even layer on a cookie sheet.

4. Bake 1 hour and 15 minutes, stirring every 10–15 minutes until toasted.

Cinnamon Toasted Butternut Squash

This side dish or snack is a great fall dish. It smells amazing and will give
you the carbohydrate boost your glycogen storage needs.

INGREDIENTS | SERVES 4

3 cups butternut squash, cubed
1 tablespoon ground cinnamon
1 teaspoon nutmeg

1. Preheat oven to 350°F.

2. Place squash in 9" × 11" baking dish. Sprinkle with cinnamon and nutmeg.

3. Bake 30 minutes or until tender and slightly brown.

Coconut-Almond Ice Cream

Even those who are not on a wheat- and dairy-free diet will love this ice cream! You can also add dairy-free carob chips (instead of chocolate chips) to this ice cream.

INGREDIENTS | SERVES 6

4 cups full-fat coconut milk

½ cup raw honey

1 tablespoon wheat-free vanilla extract

½ cup slivered almonds, toasted

No Ice Cream Maker?

What happens if you don't have an ice cream maker? Don't fret. You can easily make this without one. Add all the ingredients except almonds in a blender or food processor and blend for 2–3 minutes, until thoroughly mixed. Make sure you stop to scrape the sides of the blender too. Take the mixture out of blender and pour into an airtight freezer-safe container. Toss in almonds and stir to combine. Freeze for 6–8 hours, until it hardens.

1. Combine all the ingredients in a large mixing bowl. You might have to whisk to get the milk and honey to combine.

2. Prepare following your ice cream maker instructions. Store in the freezer for up to two weeks.

Mediterranean Green Beans

This simple recipe can be served hot or at room temperature. Add any leftovers to salads as a nice healthy addition.

INGREDIENTS | SERVES 4

1 pound fresh green beans, ends trimmed, cut into 1" pieces

2 teaspoons minced fresh rosemary

1 teaspoon lemon zest

1 tablespoon olive oil

¼ teaspoon freshly cracked black pepper

1. Fill a medium-size saucepan with cold salted water and bring to a boil over high heat. Add beans and cook until they are a vibrant green, just about 4 minutes.

2. Drain beans and transfer to a large bowl. Add remaining ingredients and toss to coat evenly. Serve warm or at room temperature.

Taking Care of Your Produce

It is best to store unwashed fresh green beans in a plastic bag in the refrigerator. When you are ready to use the beans, wash them under cold running water. Washing fruits and vegetables right before you use them keeps them fresher and prevents mold from spoiling the final product.

Roasted Kale

This is a simple recipe that yields a crisp, chewy kale that is irresistible. You can also slice up some collard greens or Swiss chard as a substitute for kale, or mix them all together for a tasty medley.

INGREDIENTS | SERVES 2

6 cups kale leaves

1 tablespoon extra-virgin olive oil

1 teaspoon garlic powder

1. Preheat oven to 375°F.

2. Place kale leaves in a medium-size bowl; toss with extra-virgin olive oil and garlic powder.

3. Roast 5 minutes; turn kale over and roast another 7–10 minutes, until kale turns brown and becomes paper-thin and brittle.

4. Remove from oven and serve immediately.

Balsamic Roasted Vegetables

This is the perfect side dish that can be made with any vegetable you have on hand. You can make double the amount and add leftover roasted vegetables to omelets—or even on top of sandwiches.

INGREDIENTS | SERVES 12

1 medium head broccoli crowns, chopped

2 medium red bell peppers, seeded and diced

1 large sweet potato, peeled and cubed

4 large carrots, peeled and chopped

1 bunch asparagus, ends trimmed and chopped

1 medium red onion, peeled and quartered

1 tablespoon chopped fresh thyme

2 tablespoons chopped fresh rosemary

3 tablespoons olive oil

3 tablespoons balsamic vinegar, divided

¼ teaspoon salt

¼ teaspoon freshly ground black pepper

1 tablespoon fresh lemon juice

1. Preheat oven to 475°F.

2. In a large bowl, combine broccoli, red bell peppers, sweet potatoes, carrots, and asparagus.

3. Separate red onion quarters into pieces, and add them to the mixture.

4. In a small bowl, stir together thyme, rosemary, oil, 2 tablespoons of balsamic vinegar, salt, and pepper. Toss with vegetables until they are coated.

5. Spread vegetables evenly on a large roasting pan. Roast 25–30 minutes, stirring every 10 minutes, or until vegetables are cooked through and browned.

6. Drizzle with fresh lemon juice and remaining 1 tablespoon balsamic vinegar.

Snow Peas with Ginger and Water Chestnuts

This is a lovely side dish that would go perfectly with an Asian-themed menu.
You could add the cooked meat of your choice to make this a full meal.

INGREDIENTS | SERVES 4

1 cup snow peas, washed

1 tablespoon olive oil

½ cup water chestnuts, rinsed
and drained

2 teaspoons fresh gingerroot, chopped

1 clove garlic, peeled and minced

Juice from ½ lemon

1 tablespoon sesame seeds

1 tablespoon wheat-free soy sauce

1. Remove strings and ends of snow peas.

2. Add olive oil to a large skillet over high heat; add peas, water chestnuts, gingerroot, garlic, lemon juice, sesame seeds, and soy sauce.

3. Continue to cook over high heat, while stirring, until peas are crisp-tender, 3–5 minutes. Serve immediately.

Basic Grilled Vegetables

These vegetables are delicious in their simplicity. But if you prefer a little more tang, sprinkle them with a little flavored oil and vinegar.

INGREDIENTS | SERVES 10

3 zucchinis, cut into ½" slices

⅛ teaspoon salt

2 eggplants, cut into ½" slices

2 bunches asparagus, stalks cut in half

1 pound button mushrooms, sliced in half

4 tablespoons butter

⅛ teaspoon ground black pepper

6 cubanelle peppers, seeded

1. Place the zucchini slices on top of two layers of paper towels. Sprinkle lightly with salt. Let sit for 10 minutes. Flip over, sprinkle with salt and let sit for another 10 minutes. Salt the eggplant the same way as the zucchini, but let rest for 20 minutes on each side.

2. Place a griddle over medium-high heat on a stovetop. Toss the asparagus and mushrooms in 1 tablespoon butter. Sprinkle them lightly with salt and pepper. Brush the grill lightly with 2 tablespoons butter. Cook the asparagus for 2–4 minutes on each side. Place them on a warmed platter.

3. Cook the mushrooms for 2–4 minutes on each side and add them to the platter. Pat the eggplant and zucchini dry and place several slices on the pan. Cook for 4–6 minutes on each side. Place them on the platter.

4. Brush both sides of the peppers with 1 tablespoon butter. Place them on the pan skin side up. Grill for 2–4 minutes on each side. Sprinkle with salt and pepper and add to the platter. Keep the platter warm until ready to serve.

Basic Sautéed Swiss Chard

Swiss chard is a hardy green with large leaves and a thick stem. It has a much milder and less-bitter taste than mustard or collard greens. Avoid leaves that are wilted, yellow, or that have holes in the spines.

INGREDIENTS | SERVES 3

1 pound Swiss chard
1 tablespoon butter
½ small onion, chopped
1 clove garlic, minced
Pinch crushed red pepper flakes
1 tablespoon cider or balsamic vinegar
⅛ teaspoon nutmeg
½ cup chicken stock
¼ teaspoon salt
¼ teaspoon ground black pepper

1. Run the chard under cold water to remove any leftover dirt. Cut the thick part of the stem out of the leaves and set aside. Tear the leaves into several pieces and place on a towel. Chop the stems into ½" pieces.

2. Place a skillet over medium heat. Once it is hot, add the butter, the stem pieces, and the onion. Cook for 5–7 minutes, or until the onion is translucent and just starting to brown.

3. Add the garlic, pepper flakes, vinegar, nutmeg, and stock. Stir to combine and bring to a boil.

4. Add the leaves and stir, cooking for 2–3 minutes before covering. They should be starting to wilt. Cook for 4–5 minutes, or until the leaves are cooked through and limp.

5. Remove the lid and stir frequently as the liquid evaporates. Taste and add more vinegar, as needed, and add salt and pepper. Serve immediately.

Tomato Pesto

Serve this fresh tomato pesto over wheat-free pasta or fresh vegetables.

INGREDIENTS | SERVES 8

2 medium tomatoes, chopped

1 large red bell pepper, seeded and chopped

2 tablespoons minced fresh parsley

2 cloves garlic

¼ cup chopped fresh basil leaves

1 tablespoon plus 1½ teaspoons rice flour

¼ teaspoon salt

⅛ teaspoon ground black pepper

2 teaspoons grated fresh raw and/or organic Parmesan cheese (optional)

1. Combine tomato, red pepper, parsley, garlic, and basil in blender. Process until finely puréed.

2. Add flour, salt, and pepper to mixture. Process in blender until thoroughly combined.

3. Transfer mixture to a heavy saucepan. Bring to a boil over medium-high heat. Reduce heat and simmer for 15 minutes.

4. Add Parmesan cheese if desired and stir well.

Storing Pesto

Most pesto freezes very well. Instead of freezing the whole batch of pesto, freeze it in portion-sized amounts in individual containers with tight-fitting lids. Skip the cheese when freezing; add it right before serving.

Romanesco with Mushroom and Wine Sauce

If you can't find romanesco you can substitute cauliflower or broccoli. If you substitute broccoli, skip the steps related to boiling the vegetable. This dish is great served over rice.

INGREDIENTS | SERVES 4

1 head romanesco
1 teaspoon salt
Water, as needed
1 pound button mushrooms, sliced
3 shallots or 1 small yellow onion, sliced
3 tablespoons butter or olive oil
½ cup port, or other heavy red wine
½ teaspoon Dijon mustard

Romanesco, a Cousin of Cabbage

The Italians call it *broccolo romanesco* and the French call it *chou romanesco*. Like broccoli and cauliflower, it is a cousin of cabbage. Pick heads that are very firm with densely packed curds. Avoid any that are more yellow than green, or that have mold on them. The stalks are inedible, but the curds can be eaten raw.

1. Rinse the romanesco and break the clusters, or curds, off the stalks. Add salt to a pot of water with a steamer basket and bring to a boil over high heat. Once the water comes to a boil, add the romanesco and cover. Cook for 5 minutes. Remove from the water and drain well.

2. Place a skillet over medium heat and add the mushrooms, shallots and butter. Cook for 10–12 minutes, stirring every few minutes, until the shallots and mushrooms have softened and browned. Add the wine and mustard and reduce the heat to low.

3. After the romanesco has drained, add it to the skillet. Cook uncovered for an additional 5–10 minutes until the romanesco has reached the desired tenderness and the wine sauce has reduced.

Kale with Bacon and Tomatoes

If you can't find kale, substitute spinach or Swiss chard and reduce the cooking time from 15 minutes to 5. You can also keep more of the bacon fat and omit the olive oil to get a truly flavorful dish. Be sure to taste the dish before adding more salt.

INGREDIENTS | SERVES 6–8

2 pounds kale

4 slices bacon

1 tablespoon butter

1 small onion, chopped

2 cloves garlic, minced

¼ teaspoon salt

¼ teaspoon ground black pepper

2 medium Roma tomatoes, seeded and chopped

2 tablespoons balsamic vinegar

All Hail Kale

Kale has been cooked in so many parts of the world, and for so long, that food historians don't know where it originated. Because it grows easily in all climates, it has migrated with travelers throughout most of the world. It's incredibly high in vitamins and minerals and has helped sustain people during rough times.

1. Strip all the stems from the leaves and discard. Wash the leaves thoroughly and shake or drain until fairly dry. Chop or tear the leaves into large pieces and set aside.

2. Place a large skillet over medium-high heat and when heated, add the strips of bacon. Cook till crisp, remove from the pan, and let cool. Pour off all but 1 tablespoon of the bacon fat.

3. Add the butter to the skillet with the bacon fat and the chopped onion. Cook for 5–7 minutes, or until the onion is soft and starting to brown. Stir in the minced garlic.

4. Add a large bunch of kale to the skillet and sprinkle with salt and pepper. Cover with a lid for 1 minute to wilt the kale. Use a spoon to move the wilted kale to the outsides of the skillet. Repeat until all of the kale has been added. Stir frequently and cook for 15–20 minutes till tender.

5. Crumble the cooked bacon and sprinkle on top with the tomato. Sprinkle the balsamic vinegar over the kale and toss to combine. Remove to a bowl and serve immediately.

Sautéed Mushrooms

Even white button mushrooms can have a lot of flavor if they're cooked right. These mushrooms can also be served over steaks, with eggs, or with polenta.

INGREDIENTS | SERVES 4

3 tablespoons butter, divided
1 pound mushrooms, sliced
½ teaspoon salt
½ teaspoon ground black pepper
4 large shallots, minced

---

1. Place a large skillet over medium heat. Add 1 tablespoon butter.

2. Add one large handful of mushrooms. Sprinkle them lightly with salt and pepper. Cook for several minutes on each side, or until they've shrunk in size and turned dark brown. Remove from skillet and keep them warm.

3. Repeat with the rest of the butter and mushrooms until all of the mushrooms are cooked.

4. If the skillet is dry, add a small amount of butter. Add the shallots and stir frequently for 5 minutes, or until they're soft and starting to brown.

5. Return the mushrooms to the skillet and stir occasionally for 3 minutes, or until the mushrooms are hot again. Serve hot.

Spicy Mustard Greens

Mustard greens are less bitter than kale or collard greens, and have a much more peppery flavor, similar to arugula. But a splash of spicy vinegar will help combat any remaining bitter flavor.

INGREDIENTS | SERVES 6

2 large bunches mustard greens
3 tablespoons butter
2 medium onions, chopped
6 cloves garlic, minced
1 teaspoon ground cumin
1 teaspoon dried crushed red pepper flakes
1 cup chicken or vegetable broth
¼ teaspoon salt
¼ teaspoon ground black pepper
Spicy vinegar, for garnish

1. Remove the veins from the mustard leaves and rinse them thoroughly in cold water. Shake dry and tear into large pieces.

2. Place a skillet over medium-high heat and once heated, add the butter and onions. Stir frequently until they're soft and starting to turn brown, about 10 minutes.

3. Stir in the garlic, cumin, and crushed red pepper and cook for 3 minutes.

4. Add one batch of the greens and cover for 1–2 minutes until the greens wilt. Repeat with the other batches until all the greens have been added and have wilted.

5. Add the broth, cover, and reduce the heat to low. Let the greens cook for 30–45 minutes. They should be very tender. Taste before adding salt and pepper. Serve while hot with spicy vinegar for people to garnish as they wish.

Blueberry, Blackberry, and Orange Salsa

The fruity aroma of this salsa will have your mouth watering. Serve it with your favorite grilled meat, chicken, or fish.

INGREDIENTS | SERVES 8

½ cup fresh blueberries, finely chopped

½ cup blackberries, finely chopped

½ jalapeño, cored, seeded, and finely chopped (optional)

1 tablespoon red onion, finely chopped

1 tablespoon chives, finely chopped

1 tablespoon cilantro, finely chopped

1 tablespoon fresh parsley, finely chopped

1 teaspoon orange zest, finely grated

1 teaspoon lemon zest, finely grated

2 tablespoons freshly squeezed orange juice

¼ teaspoon salt

¼ teaspoon ground black pepper

1. In a large mixing bowl, combine all ingredients. Mix well to combine.

2. Refrigerate and chill well before serving.

Fruit Salsas

There are many ways to get enough servings of fresh fruits, and fruit salsas are a great option! The antioxidants in the fresh blueberries and blackberries are healthy, and this recipe presents them in a unique way—a salsa!

Tomatillo Salsa

The fresh, tart, crisp flavor and green color of this salsa will blow you away! You will find yourself dipping it like guacamole.

INGREDIENTS | SERVES 12

1 cup diced tomatillos
¼ cup diced red bell pepper
¼ cup diced yellow bell pepper
¼ cup diced onion
2 tablespoons white wine vinegar
1 tablespoon lime juice
1 tablespoon lemon juice
2 teaspoons chopped fresh cilantro
½ teaspoon ground cumin
¼ teaspoon ground red pepper

I Say Tomato, You Say Tomatillo!

If you're not familiar with tomatillos, they are sometimes called the Mexican tomato or husk tomato. The fruit of the tomatillo is firm and bright green in color. Tomatillos have a papery outer skin. The flavor is tart and not like the commonly known red tomato.

1. In a large glass bowl, combine diced tomatillos, sweet red pepper, sweet yellow pepper, and onion. Mix well.

2. Fold in vinegar, lime juice, and lemon juice. Stir well to combine. Add cilantro, cumin, and ground red pepper, stirring well to combine.

3. Cover and refrigerate at least 2 hours.

4. Serve salsa with sliced vegetables. This salsa also brings out the best in cooked chicken, pork, and beef and makes for a beautiful presentation for a meal.

Lemon-Roasted Fruit

Keep adding a rainbow of fruits to your diet. This roasted fruit recipe will be a treat for an afternoon snack with a cup of tea, especially if you share it with a good friend.

INGREDIENTS | SERVES 6

2 tablespoons melted butter

2 tablespoons freshly squeezed lemon juice

1 tablespoon raw honey

3 cups pineapple chunks

6 tablespoons full-fat yogurt

Fresh mint sprigs, optional

Variations

You can substitute any fruit of your choice for the pineapple or use a variety of fruits. Peaches, pears, apples, whole strawberries, black cherries, green grapes, papaya, or mango slices all work well with this recipe. All are naturally delicious, although they are higher in sugar than berries.

1. Preheat oven to 350°F.

2. In a medium bowl, combine butter, lemon juice, and honey. Toss pineapple to coat. Let stand at room temperature for a minimum of 30 minutes or up to 2½ hours.

3. Grease a shallow glass baking dish. Place pineapple in prepared baking dish. Bake for 30 minutes or until fruit is thoroughly warmed and tender.

4. Serve cooked pineapple on individual dessert plates topped with a tablespoon of yogurt. Top with a fresh mint sprig if desired.

CHAPTER 14

Smoothies

Blueberry Antioxidant Smoothie

Blueberries contain one of the highest antioxidant levels found in fruit. This smoothie is refreshing while fighting free-radical oxidation in your body.

INGREDIENTS | SERVES 1

1 cup frozen blueberries
½ avocado
1 cup vanilla-flavored almond milk
⅛ teaspoon ground nutmeg
4–6 ice cubes

Combine all ingredients in a blender and purée until smooth.

Berry Blender Special

Super berries come together again in an almond milk-based smoothie. Creamy cashew butter adds protein and healthy fat to this treat.

INGREDIENTS | YIELDS 1½ CUPS (3 SERVINGS)

½ cup blackberries
1 cup strawberries, stems removed
½ cup raspberries
1 cup organic almond milk
1 tablespoon cashew butter
1 cup ice

Combine all ingredients in a blender and purée until smooth.

Black Raspberry-Vanilla Smoothie

*Black raspberries can be hard to find, but blending blackberries
and red raspberries together is a great substitute.*

**INGREDIENTS | YIELDS 1½ CUPS
(3 SERVINGS)**

2 cups blackberries
½ cup raspberries
1 cup full-fat vanilla yogurt
1 tablespoon raw honey

Combine all ingredients in a blender and purée
until smooth.

Brain Fuel Ice Cream

There's nothing like homemade ice cream, and this recipe is so easy, you'll never be without it!

**INGREDIENTS | YIELDS 2 CUPS
(4 SERVINGS)**

2 cups frozen berries
2 cups full-fat plain Greek yogurt
2 tablespoons raw honey

Combine all ingredients in a blender and purée until
smooth. Mixture can be refrozen in a covered container.

Raspberry Banana Smoothie

Smoothies are a wonderful, healthy, and filling alternative to standard breakfast options. They are so versatile and can be used with so many different ingredients.

INGREDIENTS | SERVES 2

1 cup plain full-fat Greek yogurt

½ cup frozen raspberries

½ cup almond milk

½ banana, peeled

2 tablespoons ground flaxseed

2 tablespoons vanilla grass-fed whey protein powder

Combine all ingredients in a blender and purée until smooth.

The Benefits of Flax

Flax is a seed that is packed with more anti-oxidants, fiber, and omega-3 fatty acids than just about anything its size. These omega-3 fatty acids are the ones that fight inflammation in the body and help prevent diseases and chronic illnesses. Ground flax-seed can be found in most supermarkets and health food stores.

Cinnamon Berry Smoothie

This smoothie is ideal for breakfast or as a snack. You can substitute different frozen fruits if you do not have frozen berries on hand.

INGREDIENTS | SERVES 2–3

2 cups almond milk

1 tablespoon raw honey

1 teaspoon wheat-free vanilla extract

½ cup frozen strawberries

½ cup frozen raspberries

1 tablespoon coconut oil

½ teaspoon cinnamon

½ cup blueberries, frozen

1 tablespoon almond butter

Combine all ingredients in a blender and purée until smooth.

A Berry Great Morning

This smoothie is packed with antioxidants, phytochemicals, and protein to get you moving and keep you moving!

INGREDIENTS | YIELDS 1 QUART (4 SERVINGS)

2 cups mixed baby greens

1 pint raspberries

1 pint blueberries

1 banana, peeled

2 tablespoons vanilla grass-fed whey protein powder

1 cup vanilla almond milk

1. Combine greens, berries, banana, and protein powder and blend thoroughly.

2. While blending, add almond milk slowly until desired texture is achieved.

Berries for a Healthy Life

Combining raspberries and blueberries in the same smoothie gives your immune system a boost. Vitamins and phytochemicals burst from these berries!

Strawberry Start

If you love strawberries, you'll be happy to enjoy one of your favorite fruits while also fulfilling your daily requirement for an entire serving of greens.

INGREDIENTS | YIELDS 3–4 CUPS

½ cup dandelion greens

2 pints strawberries

2 tablespoons vanilla grass-fed whey protein powder

1 cup vanilla almond milk

1. Add dandelion greens, strawberries, protein powder, and ½ cup almond milk in a blender and blend until combined.

2. Slowly add remaining ½ cup almond milk while blending until desired consistency is achieved.

Strawberries for Sight

Rich in the antioxidants that give them their vibrant red color, this sweet berry is also rich in vitamins A, C, D, and E, B vitamins, folate, and phytochemicals. These nutrients join forces to help you maintain healthy eyes. Strawberries may help delay the onset of macular degeneration.

Calming Cucumber

The light tastes of cucumber and spinach combine with fragrant mint in this delightfully smooth and refreshing smoothie.

INGREDIENTS | YIELDS 3–4 CUPS (3–4 SERVINGS)

1 cup spinach

2 medium cucumbers, peeled

¼ cup mint, chopped

2 tablespoons vanilla grass-fed whey protein powder

1 cup spring water

1. Place spinach, cucumbers, mint, protein powder, and ½ cup water in a blender and combine thoroughly.

2. Add remaining water while blending until desired texture is achieved.

Cucumbers and Hydration

Even though a cucumber is mostly water (and fiber), it is far more than a tasty, hydrating, and filling snack option. These green veggies are a great addition to your diet, and they're great for your skin!

The Hangover Helper

When you realize certain lifestyle choices may not make for the best days following, this smoothie is the perfect pick-me-up to calm your head and your stomach while pleasing your taste buds.

INGREDIENTS | YIELDS 3–4 CUPS (3–4 SERVINGS)

1 cup spinach

1 medium apple, cored and peeled

1 medium banana, peeled

½"–1" gingerroot, peeled and sliced or chopped

2 tablespoons vanilla grass-fed whey protein powder

1 cup vanilla almond milk

1. Place spinach, apple, banana, ginger, protein powder, and half of the almond milk in a blender and blend until thoroughly combined.

2. If needed, add remaining half of almond milk while blending until desired texture is achieved.

Ginger and Hangovers

Because the gingerroot's capabilities include alleviating symptoms associated with indigestion, nausea, and fever as well as promoting optimal blood circulation and maintaining clear sinuses, this is one ingredient that can help ease many of the symptoms resulting from an evening of too much of anything. This smoothie is a must for any of those not-so-healthy days!

Cacao Banana Smoothie

It's quite difficult to find someone who doesn't like chocolate! This smoothie has the perfect blend of ingredients to satisfy any chocolate craving.

**INGREDIENTS | YIELDS 3–4 CUPS
(3–4 SERVINGS)**

1 cup watercress

2 tablespoons raw powdered cacao

2 tablespoons chocolate grass-fed whey protein powder

2 medium bananas, peeled

2 cups almond milk

1. In a blender, place the watercress, cacao powder, and protein powder, followed by the bananas and 1 cup of the almond milk and blend until thoroughly combined.

2. Add remaining cup of almond milk while blending until desired texture is achieved.

Chocolate Is Healthy?

Chocolate has been determined to be beneficial in the daily diet! Now, don't take this as a go-ahead to dive into that huge bag of M&M's. Powdered, unprocessed cacao is the chocolate shown to provide the most benefits. Although the candy bar alternative may seem more gratifying, the sugar content, trans fats, and milk products may be the reason they haven't yet been labeled superfoods.

A Sweet Beet Treat

When you're looking for a sweet treat, beets are vitamin- and nutrient-packed vegetables that offer up a sweet earthy taste. This recipe utilizes the beet greens as well for added flavor and nutrition.

INGREDIENTS | YIELDS 3–4 CUPS (3–4 SERVINGS)

1 cup beet greens

3 medium beets

1 medium banana, peeled

2 tablespoons unflavored or vanilla grass-fed whey protein powder

1 cup almond milk

½ cup ice cubes (optional)

1. Place beet greens, beets, banana, protein powder, and ½ cup almond milk in a blender container and blend until thoroughly combined.

2. Add remaining almond milk and ice while blending until desired texture is achieved.

Beet Greens

While the actual beets are what have the reputation for being sweet, nutritious, delicious little veggies, the roots and greens of the beet are also edible and packed with calcium, potassium, and vitamins A and C.

Sinful Strawberry Cream

When a craving for something sweet and delicious hits, this is a simple go-to you're sure to enjoy. Rich, sweet, and creamy, this recipe will simultaneously satisfy your sweet tooth and supply important vitamins and minerals.

INGREDIENTS | YIELDS 3–4 CUPS (3–4 SERVINGS)

1 cup spinach

2 pints strawberries

1 medium banana, peeled

2 tablespoons grass-fed vanilla whey protein powder

1 cup kefir

1. Place spinach, strawberries, banana, protein powder, and ½ cup kefir in a blender container and blend until thoroughly combined.

2. Add remaining ½ cup kefir while blending until desired texture is achieved.

Kefir versus Milk

If you've never indulged in this awesome milk alternative, now may be the perfect time. Kefir contains a plethora of vitamins, probiotic bacteria, and enzymes that promote healthy growth, optimize digestion, and fight illness.

Pineapple Green Smoothie

The unique combination of dandelion greens, arugula, and pineapple creates a surprisingly sweet smoothie you're sure to enjoy.

INGREDIENTS | YIELDS 3–4 CUPS (3–4 SERVINGS)

½ cup dandelion greens

½ cup arugula

1 cup pineapple, peeled and cored

2 tablespoons unflavored grass-fed whey protein powder

2 cups coconut milk

1. Place dandelion greens, arugula, pineapple, protein powder, and 1 cup coconut milk in a blender and blend until thoroughly combined.

2. Add remaining 1 cup of coconut milk while blending until desired texture is achieved.

The Rich Flavors of Protein

You can easily add protein powders to your smoothies. No longer bland or chalky, protein powders are available in a wide variety of flavors and flavor combinations that will provide a healthy helping of protein while satisfying your sweet tooth. Chocolate, banana cream, and many more flavors are now available. Blend them into any smoothie recipe to increase your daily protein intake.

Cacao-Vanilla Smoothie

Bursting with flavor, this smoothie provides more nutrition than you would think. It provides a boost of vitamins, minerals, and antioxidants.

INGREDIENTS | YIELDS 3–4 CUPS (3–4 SERVINGS)

1 cup spinach

2 bananas, peeled

1 tablespoon raw cacao powder

2 tablespoons chocolate grass-fed whey protein powder

½ vanilla bean pulp

2 cups almond milk

1. Place spinach, bananas, cacao powder, protein powder, vanilla bean pulp, and 1 cup almond milk in a blender and blend until thoroughly combined.

2. Add remaining 1 cup of almond milk while blending until desired texture is achieved.

Apple and Beet Cleanser

The liver is a powerful organ responsible for removing unhealthy toxins from the body. Beet greens, beets, and apples are known to optimize liver functioning, and the addition of the banana's smooth texture makes this a healthy, tasty, liver-purifying blend.

INGREDIENTS | YIELDS 3–4 CUPS (3–4 SERVINGS)

1 cup beet greens

1 medium beet

3 medium apples, peeled and cored

1 medium banana, peeled

2 cups spring water

1. Place beet greens, beet, apples, banana, and 1 cup of water in a blender and blend until thoroughly combined.

2. Add remaining 1 cup of water as needed while blending until desired texture is achieved.

Amazing Avocados

If you're looking to add the good fats that can be found in nuts, seeds, and certain fruits to your diet, avocados should be a staple in your kitchen. The creamy texture of avocados makes a perfect addition to salads, soups, and smoothies.

**INGREDIENTS | YIELDS 3–4 CUPS
(3–4 SERVINGS)**

1 cup spinach

2 avocados, peeled and seeds removed

1 medium lime, peeled

2 tablespoons unflavored grass-fed whey protein powder

1 cup spring water

1 cup full-fat Greek-style yogurt

1. Place spinach, avocados, lime, protein powder, ½ cup water, and ½ cup yogurt in a blender and blend until thoroughly combined.

2. Add remaining ½ cup water and ½ cup yogurt while blending until desired texture is achieved.

Flaxseed in Your Smoothie

Although most of the protein powders available are sweet flavors, you can find plain ones that will add protein without altering the taste. A different type of health-benefiting addition is ground flaxseed. Rich in omega-3s and well known for regulating blood pressure, these slightly nutty-tasting seeds will boost the health benefits of your smoothie.

Alcohol Recovery Recipe

Although this smoothie may not relieve that pounding headache, it will definitely assist your liver in flushing out the toxins provided by alcohol consumption. This delightful blend will get your body back on track!

INGREDIENTS | YIELDS 3–4 CUPS (3–4 SERVINGS)

1 cup spinach

3 medium carrots, peeled

2 medium apples, peeled and cored

1 medium beet

2½ cups spring water

1. Place spinach, carrots, apples, beet, and half of the water in a blender and blend until thoroughly combined.

2. Add remaining half of the water as needed while blending until desired texture is achieved.

Combating the Effects of Alcohol

Because alcohol can really do a number on your liver, it is important to supply your body with the best foods to maintain your liver's optimal functioning following heavy alcohol consumption. Spinach, carrots, apples, beets, lemon, wheatgrass, and grapefruit have shown to be true super-foods when it comes to purging the liver of harmful toxins. In addition, they are also high in vitamin C and promote health while minimizing feelings of moodiness and depression.

Cleansing Green Smoothie

The ingredients in this smoothie will help you cleanse your gallbladder. Responsible for removing toxins and waste from the body along with the liver, the gallbladder is an important part of the body's makeup.

INGREDIENTS | YIELDS 3–4 CUPS (3–4 SERVINGS)

1 cup spinach

1 cup asparagus spears

½ medium lemon, peeled

1 medium tomato

1–2 cloves garlic, depending upon size

2 cups spring water

1. Place spinach, asparagus, lemon, tomato, garlic, and 1 cup water in a blender and blend until thoroughly combined.

2. Add remaining 1 cup of water as needed while blending until desired texture is achieved.

Why Does Gallbladder Health Matter?

Bile acids made in the liver and used by the small intestine for breaking down foods in digestion are stored in the gallbladder. If the gallbladder isn't functioning properly, digestion can be a difficult and painful process. By promoting a healthy gallbladder, you're ensuring the digestive process moves as smoothly and regularly as possible.

Blackberry-Ginger-Lemon Green Smoothie

Delicious blackberries are made even more tasty with the addition of lemon and ginger in this recipe. This smoothie packs a healthy dose of much-needed vitamins and minerals, and is rich and satisfying with the addition of protein-packed yogurt.

**INGREDIENTS | YIELDS 3–4 CUPS
(3–4 SERVINGS)**

1 cup watercress

2 pints blackberries

1 medium banana, peeled

½ medium lemon, peeled

½" slice gingerroot, peeled

1 cup full-fat Greek-style yogurt

1. Place watercress, blackberries, banana, lemon, gingerroot, and ½ cup of yogurt in a blender and blend until thoroughly combined.

2. Add remaining ½ cup yogurt as needed while blending until desired consistency is achieved.

Blackberries Promote Respiratory Relief

Rich blackberries are not just a tasty treat, they are also packed with a variety of vitamins and minerals that can aid in overall health. Specifically, the magnesium content in blackberries is what makes it a crusader in promoting respiratory ease. Best known for its ability to relax the muscles and thin mucus most commonly associated with breathing difficulties, blackberries are an important addition to those in need of breathing assistance.

Luscious Lemon Smoothie

Lemon is a refreshing ingredient and is packed with vitamin C. Not only does this vitamin aid in building immunity, it plays an important role in the metabolism of fat!

INGREDIENTS | YIELDS 3–4 CUPS (3–4 SERVINGS)

1 cup watercress
2 medium lemons, peeled
2 medium cucumbers, peeled
½" slice gingerroot, peeled
2 cups spring water

1. Place watercress, lemons, cucumbers, gingerroot, and 1 cup of water in a blender and blend until thoroughly combined.

2. Add remaining 1 cup of water as needed while blending until desired consistency is achieved.

Ginger-Berry Smoothie

Antioxidant-rich blueberries and fat-burning blackberries pair up with soothing ginger for a refreshingly light smoothie.

INGREDIENTS | YIELDS 3–4 CUPS (3–4 SERVINGS)

1 cup watercress
2 cups blueberries
1 cup blackberries
½" slice gingerroot, peeled
2 cups green tea

1. Place watercress, berries, gingerroot, and 1 cup tea in a blender and blend until thoroughly combined.

2. Add remaining 1 cup of green tea as needed while blending until desired consistency is achieved.

Magic Berries

Blueberries, blackberries, strawberries, and raspberries are superfoods disguised as sweet treats. These fat-burning fruits are low in calories, packed with antioxidants that promote weight loss, and supply quick energy that also allows you to burn fat fast.

Green Tea Metabolism Booster

Green tea is packed with fat-burning catechin antioxidants that aid in weight loss. Using green tea instead of water in this smoothie amplifies the fat-burning properties of the vitamin- and mineral-rich greens and fruits.

INGREDIENTS | YIELDS 3–4 CUPS (3–4 SERVINGS)

1 cup watercress

1 medium lemon, peeled

2 cups cantaloupe, rind and seeds removed

1 cup raspberries

2 cups green tea

1. Place watercress, lemon, cantaloupe, raspberries, and 1 cup of tea in a blender and blend until thoroughly combined.

2. Add remaining 1 cup of tea as needed while blending until desired consistency is achieved.

Making Quick Green Tea

Most people who are on the go prefer to make their green tea with the conveniently prepackaged tea bags. By purchasing quality green tea bags and using quality spring water, you can make your own fat-burning green tea on the go, at the office, or even in the car. Boil the water and pour it into a safe (preferably glass) container, steep the tea bag for the suggested amount of time to maximize antioxidant release and taste, and enjoy!

Refreshing Fruit Smoothie

When you're feeling dried out, tired, or just down, vitamin C–rich smoothies like this one can give you automatic energy that will pick you up and keep you going.

INGREDIENTS | YIELDS 3–4 CUPS (SERVES 3–4)

1 cup watercress
½ cantaloupe, rind and seeds removed
1 cup strawberries
1 medium orange, peeled
½ medium lemon, peeled
1 cup green tea

1. Place watercress, cantaloupe, strawberries, orange, lemon, and ½ cup of tea in a blender and blend until thoroughly combined.

2. Add remaining green tea as needed while blending until desired consistency is achieved.

Vitamin C Deficiencies

Even though orange juice, fresh produce, and affordable fruits and vegetables packed with vitamin C are readily available and accessible to Americans, most don't get the recommended daily value of 60 mg per day. Although multivitamins and vitamin C pill alternatives provide loads of vitamin C, the fresh sources of this important vitamin are a healthier, more refreshing option that can give you the added benefits of extra vitamins and minerals.

Tropical Green Smoothie

This smoothie is packed with vitamin C. Vitamin C is an important addition to your diet for its immunity-building power, and it helps promote optimal brain functioning, which means better mental clarity and improved focus.

INGREDIENTS | YIELDS 3–4 CUPS (SERVES 3–4)

1 cup watercress
2 medium tangerines, peeled
½ medium grapefruit, peeled
½ pineapple, peeled and cored
½ cantaloupe, rind and seeds removed
1 cup red raspberry tea

1. Place watercress, tangerines, grapefruit, pineapple, and cantaloupe in a blender and blend until thoroughly combined.

2. Add 1 cup of tea as needed while blending until desired consistency is achieved.

Green Tea Green Smoothie

Intense nutrition is packed into a green smoothie. Antioxidant-rich green tea blends with vitamin- and mineral-packed spinach, ginger, and lemon.

INGREDIENTS | YIELDS 3–4 CUPS

1 cup spinach
2 medium lemons, peeled
½" slice gingerroot, peeled
1 tablespoon raw honey
2 cups green tea

1. Place spinach, lemons, ginger, honey, and 1 cup of tea in a blender and blend until thoroughly combined.

2. Add remaining 1 cup of tea as needed while blending until desired consistency is achieved.

APPENDIX A

Resources

Not Just Paleo

Evan Brand's Website
www.notjustpaleo.com

Evan Brand's Store: Recommended Products
www.notjustpaleo.com/resources

Functional Lab Testing
www.im.notjustpaleo.com/shop

Products

Free Blue-Light-Blocking Software
www.justgetflux.com

www.douglaslabs.com

www.onnit.com
(use *www.notjustpaleo.com/supplements* for
10% discount at Onnit)

www.veropure.com

www.thorne.com

www.bulletproofexec.com

Recommended Reading

The Edge Effect by Dr. Eric Braverman

The Diet Cure by Julia Ross

The Ultramind Solution by Dr. Mark Hyman

DMT: The Spirit Molecule by Dr. Rick Strassman

Nutrition and Physical Degeneration by Weston A.
Price, DDS

Nutrient Power by William Walsh, PhD

Why Stomach Acid Is Good for You by Jonathan
Wright, MD

Lights Out by T.S. Wiley

Do The Work by Steven Pressfield

APPENDIX B

Bibliography

Chapter 2

aan het Rot, Benkelfat, Boivin, and Young. 2008. "Bright light exposure during acute tryptophan depletion prevents a lowering of mood in mildly seasonal women." *European Neuropsychopharmacology. www.ncbi.nlm.nih .gov/pubmed/17582745/*

aan het Rot, Moskowitz, and Young. 2008. "Exposure to bright light is associated with positive social interaction and good mood over short time periods: A naturalistic study in mildly seasonal people." *Journal of Psychiatric Research. www.ncbi.nlm.nih.gov/pubmed/17275841/*

Audero, Coppi, Mlinar, Rossetti, Caprioli, Banchaabouchi, Corradetti, and Gross. 2008. "Sporadic autonomic dysregulation and death associated with excessive serotonin autoinhibition." *Science. www.ncbi.nlm.nih.gov/ pubmed/18599790*

Benmansour, Cecchi, Morilak, Gerhardt, Javors, Gould, and Frazer. 1999. "Effects of chronic antidepressant treatments on serotonin transporter function, density, and mRNA level." *Journal of Neuroscience. www.ncbi.nlm .nih.gov/pubmed/10575045*

Berridge and Devilbiss. 2011. "Psychostimulants as cognitive enhancers: the prefrontal cortex, catecholamines, and attention-deficit/hyperactivity disorder." *Biological Psychiatry. www.ncbi.nlm.nih.gov/pubmed/20875636*

Ferraro and Steger. 1990. "Diurnal variations in brain serotonin are driven by the photic cycle and are not circadian in nature." *Brain Research. www.ncbi.nlm.nih.gov/pubmed/2337799/*

Platt and Reidel. 2011. "The cholinergic system, EEG and sleep." *Behavioural Brain Research. www.ncbi.nlm.nih.gov/pubmed/21238497*

Salmon. 2001. "Effects of physical exercise on anxiety, depression, and sensitivity to stress: a unifying theory." *Clinical Psychology Review. www.ncbi.nlm.nih.gov/pubmed/11148895/*

Chapter 4

Croisile, Trillet, Fondarai, Laurent, Mauguière, and Billardon. 1993. "Long-term and high-dose piracetam treatment of Alzheimer's disease." *Neurology. www.ncbi.nlm.nih.gov/pubmed/8437693*

Malykh and Sadaie. 2010. "Piracetam and piracetam-like drugs: from basic science to novel clinical applications to CNS disorders." *Drugs. www.ncbi .nlm.nih.gov/pubmed/20166767*

Chapter 5

Arnold, Feifel, Earl, Yang, and Adler. 2014. "A 9-week, randomized, double-blind, placebo-controlled, parallel-group, dose-finding study to evaluate the efficacy and safety of modafinil as treatment for adults with ADHD." *Journal of Attention Disorders. www.ncbi.nlm.nih.gov/pubmed/22617860*

Banderet and Lieberman. 1989. "Treatment with tyrosine, a neurotransmitter precursor, reduces environmental stress in humans." *Brain Research Bulletin. www.ncbi.nlm.nih.gov/pubmed/2736402*

Baumel, Eisner, Karukin, MacNamara, Katz, and Deveaugh-Geiss. 1989. "Oxiracetam in the treatment of multi-infarct dementia." *Progress in Neuropsychopharmacology and Biological Psychiatry. www.ncbi.nlm.nih .gov/pubmed/2781039*

Copani, Genazzani, Aleppo, Casabona, Canonico, Scapagnini, and Nicoletti. 1992. "Nootropic drugs positively modulate alpha-amino-3-hydroxy-5-methyl-4-isoxazolepropionic acid-sensitive glutamate receptors in neuronal cultures." *Journal of Neurochemistry. www.ncbi.nlm.nih.gov/ pubmed/1372342*

Corasaniti, Paoletti, Palma, Granato, Navarra, and Nisticò. 1995. "Systemic administration of pramiracetam increases nitric oxide synthase activity in the cerebral cortex of the rat." *Functional Neurology. www.ncbi.nlm.nih .gov/pubmed/8557218*

Deijen, Wientjes, Vullinghs, Cloin, and Langefeld. 1999. "Tyrosine improves cognitive performance and reduces blood pressure in cadets after one week of a combat training course." *Brain Research Bulletin. www.ncbi.nlm .nih.gov/pubmed/10230711*

Dysken, Katz, Stallone, and Kuskowski. 1989. "Oxiracetam in the treatment of multi-infarct dementia and primary degenerative dementia." *Journal of Neuropsychiatry and Clinical Neurosciences. www.ncbi.nlm.nih.gov/ pubmed/2521069*

Ghelardini, Galeotti, Gualtieri, Romanelli, Bucherelli, Baldi, and Bartolini. 2002. "DM235 (sunifiram): a novel nootropic with potential as a cognitive enhancer." *Naunyn Schmiedebergs Archives of Pharmacology. www.ncbi .nlm.nih.gov/pubmed/12070754*

Itil, Menon, Bozak, and Songar. 1982. "The effects of oxiracetam (ISF 2522) in patients with organic brain syndrome (a double-blind controlled study with piracetam)." *Drug Development Research. http://onlinelibrary.wiley .com/doi/10.1002/ddr.430020506/abstract*

Knapp, Goldenberg, Shuck, Cecil, Watkins, Miller, Crites, and Malatynska. 2002. "Antidepressant activity of memory-enhancing drugs in the reduction of submissive behavior model." *European Journal of Pharmacology. www .ncbi.nlm.nih.gov/pubmed/11959085*

Koval'chuk, V.V., Skoromets, Koval'chuk, I.V., Stoianova, Vysotskaia, Melikhova, and Il'iainen. 2010. "Efficacy of phenotropil in the rehabilitation of stroke patients." *Zh Nevrol Psikhiatr Im S S Korsakova* (article in Russian). *www.ncbi.nlm.nih.gov/pubmed/21626817*

Kraemer, Volek, French, Rubin, Sharman, Gomez, Ratamess, Newton, Jemiolo, Craig, and Häkkinen. 2003. "The effects of L-carnitine L-tartrate supplementation on hormonal responses to resistance exercise and recovery." *The Journal of Strength and Conditioning Research. www.ncbi .nlm.nih.gov/pubmed/12930169*

Lee and Benfield. 1994. "Aniracetam. An overview of its pharmacodynamic and pharmacokinetic properties, and a review of its therapeutic potential in senile cognitive disorders." *Drugs & Aging. www.ncbi.nlm.nih.gov/pubmed/8199398*

Malaguarnera, M., Vacante, Motta, Giordano, Malaguarnera, G., Bella, Nunnari, Rampello, and Pennisi. 2011. "Acetyl-L-carnitine improves cognitive functions in severe hepatic encephalopathy: a randomized and controlled clinical trial." *Metabolic Brain Disease. www.ncbi.nlm.nih.gov/pubmed/21870121*

Mauri, Sinforiani, Reverberi, Merlo, and Bono. 1994. "Pramiracetam effects on scopolamine-induced amnesia in healthy volunteers." *Archives of Gerontology and Geriatrics. www.ncbi.nlm.nih.gov/pubmed/15374306*

McLean, Cardenas, Burgess, and Gamzu. 1991. "Placebo-controlled study of pramiracetam in young males with memory and cognitive problems resulting from head injury and anoxia." *Brain Injury. www.ncbi.nlm.nih.gov/pubmed/1786500*

Mordyk, Lysov, Kondria, Gol'dzon, and Khlebova. 2009. "Prevention of neuro- and cardiotoxic side effects of tuberculosis chemotherapy with noopept." *Klinicheskaia meditsina* (article in Russian). *www.ncbi.nlm.nih.gov/pubmed/19565831*

Neri, Wiegmann, Stanny, Shappell, McCardie, and McKay. 1995. "The effects of tyrosine on cognitive performance during extended wakefulness." *Aviation, Space, and Environmental Medicine. www.ncbi.nlm.nih.gov/pubmed/7794222*

Pigeau, Naitoh, Buguet, McCann, Baranski, Taylor, Thompson, and MacK. 1995. "Modafinil, d-amphetamine and placebo during 64 hours of sustained mental work. I. Effects on mood, fatigue, cognitive performance and body temperature." *Journal of Sleep Research. www.ncbi.nlm.nih.gov/pubmed/10607161*

Ruggenenti, Cattaneo, Loriga, Ledda, Motterlini, Gherardi, Orisio, and Remuzzi. 2009. "Ameliorating hypertension and insulin resistance in subjects at increased cardiovascular risk: effects of acetyl-L-carnitine therapy." *Hypertension. www.ncbi.nlm.nih.gov/pubmed/19620516*

Savchenko, Zakharova, and Stepanov. 2005. "The phenotropil treatment of the consequences of brain organic lesions." *Zh Nevrol Psikhiatr Im S S Korsakova* (article in Russian). *www.ncbi.nlm.nih.gov/pubmed/16447562*

Smart, Desmond, Poulos, and Zack. 2013. "Modafinil increases reward salience in a slot machine game in low and high impulsivity pathological gamblers." *Neuropharmacology. www.ncbi.nlm.nih.gov/pubmed/23711549*

Taupin. 2009. "Nootropic agents stimulate neurogenesis." *Expert Opinion on Therapeutic Patents. www.ncbi.nlm.nih.gov/pubmed/19441945*

Volek, Kraemer, Rubin, Gómez, Ratamess, and Gaynor. 2002. "L-Carnitine L-tartrate supplementation favorably affects markers of recovery from exercise stress." *American Journal of Physiology, Endocrinology and Metabolism. www.ncbi.nlm.nih.gov/pubmed/11788381*

Watanabe, Kono, Nakashima, Mitsunobu, and Otsuki. 1975. "Effects of various cerebral metabolic activators on glucose metabolism of brain." *Japanese Journal of Psychiatry and Neurology. www.ncbi.nlm.nih.gov/pubmed/1098982*

Chapter 7

Barbagallo, S.G., Barbagallo, M., Giordano, Meli, and Panzarasa. 1994. "alpha-Glycerophosphocholine in the mental recovery of cerebral ischemic attacks. An Italian multicenter clinical trial." *Annals of the New York Academy of Sciences. www.ncbi.nlm.nih.gov/pubmed/8030842*

Benton and Donohoe. 2011. "The influence of creatine supplementation on the cognitive functioning of vegetarians and omnivores." *British Journal of Nutrition. www.ncbi.nlm.nih.gov/pubmed/21118604*

Conant and Schauss. 2004. "Therapeutic applications of citicoline for stroke and cognitive dysfunction in the elderly: a review of the literature." *Alternative Medicine Review. www.ncbi.nlm.nih.gov/pubmed/15005642*

Cotroneo, Castagna, Putignano, Lacava, Fantò, Monteleone, Rocca, Malara, and Gareri. 2013. "Effectiveness and safety of citicoline in mild vascular cognitive impairment: the IDEALE study." *Clinical Interventions in Aging. www.ncbi.nlm.nih.gov/pubmed/23403474*

De Jesus Moreno. 2003. "Cognitive improvement in mild to moderate Alzheimer's dementia after treatment with the acetylcholine precursor choline alfoscerate: a multicenter, double-blind, randomized, placebo-controlled trial." *Clinical Therapeutics. www.ncbi.nlm.nih.gov/pubmed/12637119*

Einöther, Martens, Rycroft, and De Bruin. 2010. "L-theanine and caffeine improve task switching but not intersensory attention or subjective alertness." *Appetite. www.ncbi.nlm.nih.gov/pubmed/20079786*

Glade and Smith. 2015. "Phosphatidylserine and the human brain." *Nutrition. www.ncbi.nlm.nih.gov/pubmed/25933483*

Gomez-Ramirez, Higgins, Rycroft, Owen, Mahoney, Shpaner, and Foxe. 2007. "The deployment of intersensory selective attention: a high-density electrical mapping study of the effects of theanine." *Clinical Neuropharmacology. www.ncbi.nlm.nih.gov/pubmed/17272967*

Grieb. 2014. "Neuroprotective properties of citicoline: facts, doubts and unresolved issues." *CNS Drugs. www.ncbi.nlm.nih.gov/pubmed/24504829*

Hellhammer, Vogt, Franz, Freitas, and Rutenberg. 2014. "A soy-based phosphatidylserine/phosphatidic acid complex (PAS) normalizes the stress reactivity of hypothalamus-pituitary-adrenal-axis in chronically stressed male subjects: a randomized, placebo-controlled study." *Lipids in Health and Disease. www.ncbi.nlm.nih.gov/pubmed/25081826*

Hirayama, S., Terasawa, Rabeler, Hirayama, T., Inoue, Tatsumi, Purpura, and Jäger. 2014. "The effect of phosphatidylserine administration on memory and symptoms of attention-deficit hyperactivity disorder: a randomised, double-blind, placebo-controlled clinical trial." *Journal of Human Nutrition and Dietetics. www.ncbi.nlm.nih.gov/pubmed/23495677*

Kingsley, Wadsworth, Kilduff, McEneny, and Benton. 2005. "Effects of phosphatidylserine on oxidative stress following intermittent running." *Medicine and Science in Sports & Exercise. www.ncbi.nlm.nih.gov/pubmed/16118575*

Rae, Digney, McEwan, and Bates. 2003. "Oral creatine monohydrate supplementation improves brain performance: a double-blind, placebo-controlled, cross-over trial." *Proceedings of the Royal Society B: Biological Sciences. www.ncbi.nlm.nih.gov/pubmed/14561278*

Richter, Herzog, Lifshitz, Hayun, and Zchut. 2013. "The effect of soybean-derived phosphatidylserine on cognitive performance in elderly with subjective memory complaints: a pilot study." *Clinical Interventions in Aging. www.ncbi.nlm.nih.gov/pubmed/23723695*

Starks, M.A., Starks, S.L., Kingsley, Purpura, and Jäger. 2008. "The effects of phosphatidylserine on endocrine response to moderate intensity exercise." *Journal of the International Society of Sports Nutrition. www.ncbi.nlm.nih.gov/pubmed/18662395*

Unno, Tanida, Ishii, Yamamoto, Iguchi, Hoshino, Takeda, Ozawa, Ohkubo, Juneja, and Yamada. 2013. "Anti-stress effect of theanine on students during pharmacy practice: positive correlation among salivary α-amylase activity, trait anxiety and subjective stress." *Pharmacology, Biochemistry, and Behavior. www.ncbi.nlm.nih.gov/pubmed/24051231*

Yoto, Motoki, Murao, and Yokogoshi. 2012. "Effects of L-theanine or caffeine intake on changes in blood pressure under physical and psychological stresses." *Journal of Physiological Anthropology. www.ncbi.nlm.nih.gov/pubmed/23107346*

Chapter 8

Amieva, Meillon, Helmer, Barberger-Gateau, and Dartigues. 2013. "Ginkgo biloba extract and long-term cognitive decline: a 20-year follow-up population-based study." *PLoS One. www.ncbi.nlm.nih.gov/pubmed/23326356*

Chen, Li, Krochmal, Abrazado, Kim, and Cooper. 2010. "Effect of Cs-4 (Cordyceps sinensis) on exercise performance in healthy older subjects: a double-blind, placebo-controlled trial." *Journal of Alternative and Complementary Medicine. www.ncbi.nlm.nih.gov/pubmed/20804368*

Ginkgo Pages, The. "A-bombed Ginkgo trees in Hiroshima, Japan." *http://kwanten.home.xs4all.nl/hiroshima.htm*

Hwang, Lim, Yoo, Lee, Kim, Kang, Kwon, Park, Choi, and Won. 2008. "A Phytochemically characterized extract of Cordyceps militaris and cordycepin protect hippocampal neurons from ischemic injury in gerbils." *Planta Medica. www.ncbi.nlm.nih.gov/pubmed/18214814*

Kalman, Feldman, S., Feldman, R., Schwartz, Krieger, and Garrison. 2008. "Effect of a proprietary Magnolia and Phellodendron extract on stress levels in healthy women: a pilot, double-blind, placebo-controlled clinical trial." *Nutrition Journal. www.ncbi.nlm.nih.gov/pubmed/18426577*

Nagano, Shimizu, Kondo, Hayashi, Sato, Kitagawa, and Ohnuki. 2010. "Reduction of depression and anxiety by 4 weeks Hericium erinaceus intake." *Biomedical Research. www.ncbi.nlm.nih.gov/pubmed/20834180*

Ogunrin. 2014. "Effect of vinpocetine (cognitol™) on cognitive performances of a nigerian population." *Annals of Medical and Health Sciences Research. www.ncbi.nlm.nih.gov/pubmed/25221724*

Talbott, S.M., Talbott, J.A., and Pugh. 2013. "Effect of Magnolia officinalis and Phellodendron amurense (Relora®) on cortisol and psychological mood state in moderately stressed subjects." *Journal of the International Society of Sports Nutrition. www.ncbi.nlm.nih.gov/pubmed/23924268*

Uebel-von Sandersleben, Rothenberger, A., Albrecht, Rothenberger, L.G., Klement, and Bock. 2014. "Ginkgo biloba extract EGb 761® in children with ADHD." *Zeitschrift für Kinder- und Jugendpsychiatrie und Psychotherapie* (article in German). *www.ncbi.nlm.nih.gov/pubmed/25163996*

University of Maryland Medical Center. 2013. "Ginkgo biloba." *http://umm .edu/health/medical/altmed/herb/ginkgo-biloba*

Valikovics, Csányi, and Németh. 2012. "Study of the effects of vinpocetin on cognitive functions." *Ideggyógyászati szemle* (article in Hungarian). *www.ncbi.nlm.nih.gov/pubmed/23136730*

Wang, Zhang, and Zhan. 2006. "Effect of huperzine A on cerebral cholinesterase and acetylcholine in elderly patients during recovery from general anesthesia." *Nan Fang Yi Ke Da Xue Xue Bao* (article in Chinese). *www.ncbi.nlm.nih.gov/pubmed/17121726*

Wong, Kanagasabapathy, Naidu, David, and Sabaratnam. 2014. "Hericium erinaceus (Bull.: Fr.) Pers., a medicinal mushroom, activates peripheral nerve regeneration." *Chinese Journal of Integrative Medicine. www.ncbi.nlm .nih.gov/pubmed/25159861*

Xu, Liang, Juan-Wu, Zhang, Zhu, and Jiang. 2012. "Treatment with Huperzine A improves cognition in vascular dementia patients." *Cell Biochemistry and Biophysics. www.ncbi.nlm.nih.gov/pubmed/21833673*

Chapter 9

Agarwa, Sharma, Fatima, and Jain. 2014. "An update on Ayurvedic herb *Convolvulus pluricaulis* Choisy." *Asian Pacific Journal of Tropical Biomedicine. www.ncbi.nlm.nih.gov/pmc/articles/PMC3868798/*

Auf'mkolk, Ingbar, Kubota, Amir, and Ingbar. 1985. "Extracts and auto-oxidized constituents of certain plants inhibit the receptor-binding and the biological activity of Graves' immunoglobulins." *Endocrinology. www.ncbi .nlm.nih.gov/pubmed/2985357*

Banerjee and Izquierdo. 1982. "Antistress and antifatigue properties of Panax ginseng: comparison with piracetam." *Acta physiologica latino americana. www.ncbi.nlm.nih.gov/pubmed/6892267*

Bradwejn, Zhou, Koszycki, and Shlik. 2000. "A double-blind, placebo-controlled study on the effects of Gotu Kola (Centella asiatica) on acoustic startle response in healthy subjects." *Journal of Clinical Psychopharmacology. www.ncbi.nlm.nih.gov/pubmed/11106141*

Cayer, Ahmed, Filion, Saleem, Cuerrier, Allard, Rochefort, Merali, and Arnason. 2013. "Characterization of the anxiolytic activity of Nunavik Rhodiola rosea." *Planta Medica. www.ncbi.nlm.nih.gov/pubmed/23975866*

Chengappa, Bowie, Schlicht, Fleet, Brar, and Jindal. 2013. "Randomized placebo-controlled adjunctive study of an extract of withania somnifera for cognitive dysfunction in bipolar disorder." *Journal of Clinical Psychiatry. www.ncbi.nlm.nih.gov/pubmed/24330893*

Darbre, Bakir, and Iskakova. 2013. "Effect of aluminium on migratory and invasive properties of MCF-7 human breast cancer cells in culture." *Journal of Inorganic Biochemistry. www.ncbi.nlm.nih.gov/pubmed/23896199*

Dhuley. 2001. "Nootropic-like effect of ashwagandha (Withania somnifera L.) in mice." *Phytotherapy Research. www.ncbi.nlm.nih.gov/pubmed/11536383*

Edwards, Heufelder, and Zimmermann. 2012. "Therapeutic effects and safety of Rhodiola rosea extract WS® 1375 in subjects with life-stress symptoms—results of an open-label study." *Phytotherapy Research. www.ncbi.nlm.nih.gov/pubmed/22228617*

Fintelmann and Gruenwald. 2007. "Efficacy and tolerability of a Rhodiola rosea extract in adults with physical and cognitive deficiencies." *Advances in Therapy. www.ncbi.nlm.nih.gov/pubmed/17901042*

Kennedy, Little, and Scholey. 2004. "Attenuation of laboratory-induced stress in humans after acute administration of Melissa officinalis (Lemon Balm)." *Psychosomatic Medicine. www.ncbi.nlm.nih.gov/pubmed/15272110*

Neale, Camfield, Reay, Stough, and Scholey. 2013. "Cognitive effects of two nutraceuticals Ginseng and Bacopa benchmarked against modafinil: a review and comparison of effect sizes." *British Journal of Clinical Pharmacology. www.ncbi.nlm.nih.gov/pubmed/23043278*

Niederhofer. 2009. "First preliminary results of an observation of Panax ginseng treatment in patients with autistic disorder." *Journal of Dietary Supplements. www.ncbi.nlm.nih.gov/pubmed/22435515*

Noreen, Buckley, Lewis, Brandauer, and Stuempfle. 2013. "The effects of an acute dose of Rhodiola rosea on endurance exercise performance." *The Journal of Strength and Conditioning Research. www.ncbi.nlm.nih.gov/ pubmed/23443221*

Reay, Scholey, and Kennedy. 2010. "Panax ginseng (G115) improves aspects of working memory performance and subjective ratings of calmness in healthy young adults." *Human Psychopharmacology. www.ncbi.nlm.nih .gov/pubmed/20737519*

Scholey, Ossoukhova, Owen, Ibarra, Pipingas, He, Roller, and Stough. 2010. "Effects of American ginseng (Panax quinquefolius) on neurocognitive function: an acute, randomised, double-blind, placebo-controlled, crossover study." *Psychopharmacology. www.ncbi.nlm.nih.gov/ pubmed/20676609*

Sengupta, Toh, Sellers, Skepper, Koolwijk, Leung, Yeung, Wong, Sasisekharan, and Fan. 2004. "Modulating angiogenesis: the yin and the yang in ginseng." *Circulation. www.ncbi.nlm.nih.gov/pubmed/15337705*

Thomas, Joy, Ajayan, and Paulose. 2013. "Neuroprotective potential of Bacopa monnieri and Bacoside A against dopamine receptor dysfunction in the cerebral cortex of neonatal hypoglycaemic rats." *Cellular and Molecular Neurobiology. www.ncbi.nlm.nih.gov/pubmed/23975094*

USDA Natural Resources Conservation Service. 2015. *"Melissa officinalis* L. common balm." *http://plants.usda.gov/core/profile?symbol=MEOF2*

Van Kampen, Baranowski, Shaw, and Kay. 2014. "Panax ginseng is neuroprotective in a novel progressive model of Parkinson's disease." *Experimental Gerontology. www.ncbi.nlm.nih.gov/pubmed/24316034*

Wattanathorn, Mator, Muchimapura, Tongun, Pasuriwong, Piyawatkul, Yimtae, Sripanidkulchai, and Singkhoraard. 2008. "Positive modulation of cognition and mood in the healthy elderly volunteer following the administration of Centella asiatica." *Journal of Ethnopharmacology. www.ncbi.nlm.nih.gov/pubmed/18191355*

Yoo, D.Y., Choi, Kim, Yoo, K.Y., Lee, Yoon, Won, and Hwang. 2011. "Effects of Melissa officinalis L. (lemon balm) extract on neurogenesis associated with serum corticosterone and GABA in the mouse dentate gyrus." *Neurochemical Research. www.ncbi.nlm.nih.gov/pubmed/21076869*

Yue, Mak, Cheng, Leung, Ng, Fan, Yeung, and Wong. 2007. "Pharmacogenomics and the Yin/Yang actions of ginseng: anti-tumor, angiomodulating and steroid-like activities of ginsenosides." *Chinese Medicine. www.cmjournal.org/content/2/1/6*

Zeraatpishe, Oryan, Bagheri, Pilevarian, Malekirad, Baeeri, and Abdollahi. 2011. "Effects of Melissa officinalis L. on oxidative status and DNA damage in subjects exposed to long-term low-dose ionizing radiation." *Toxicology and Industrial Health. www.ncbi.nlm.nih.gov/pubmed/20858648*

APPENDIX C

Glossary

Acetylcholine

The first neurotransmitter to be identified. It plays an important role in both memory and learning.

Adaptogens

A category of plants, herbs, nutrients, or other compounds that help the body adapt to various forms of stress

Adrafinil

A compound that decreases your ability to sleep, and has been shown to induce orofacial dyskinesia

Adrenal glands

Endocrine glands located on top of each kidney. The adrenal glands are responsible for secreting steroid hormones and epinephrine and norepinephrine.

Adrenaline

A hormone excreted by the adrenal glands in times of stress

Alpha-GPC

A choline supplement that can be delivered across the blood-brain barrier

Aniracetam

A supplement that helps alleviate damage done to memory and learning impairments due to trauma or other cognitive impairments

Anxiolytics

Nootropics that help ease anxiety

Ashwagandha

An adaptogenic herb that helps with adrenal fatigue, sleep, and burnout. It rejuvenates the body.

Ayurveda

A system of natural healing that has been used for 5,000 years

Bacopa monnieri

An herb used as a cognitive enhancer in Ayurveda medicine. It helps protect dopamine receptor dysfunction in the brain, which helps maintain your energy and drive.

Blood brain barrier

A highly selective barrier that, when intact, prevents toxins from entering the brain

Blood sugar

The concentration of glucose in your blood

Carnitine

A combination of amino acids lysine and methionine that are produced by your liver and kidneys

Centrophenoxine

A drug used to treat Alzheimer's disease and help with symptoms of senility

Choline

An essential nutrient in the B-vitamin family

Cholinergics

A substance that interacts with the acetylcholine system

Citocoline

A naturally occurring compound that is necessary for the synthesis of phosphatidylcholine, an important phospholipid for the brain. It is made up of choline and cytidine, which are readily absorbed by the gastrointestinal tract and blood-brain barrier.

Cordyceps sinensis

A medicinal mushroom that has been used to improve performance

Cortisol

A stress hormone that combines with other hormones to pump blood to the extremities to allow faster running, stronger arms, and a general heightened sense of awareness

Creatine

A naturally occurring chemical that supplies energy to all cells in the body

Dopamine

A neurotransmitter linked to pleasure, reward, drive, and personal motivation

Enzymes

A substance produced by a living organism that prompts a biochemical reaction

Epinephrine

Another term for adrenaline

GABA (gamma-aminobutyric acid)

A chemical produced in the brain that inhibits the activation of neurons

Ginkgo biloba

A tree whose leaves improve memory and cognitive function

Gotu Kola

A wound healing and blood purifying herb that recent research has found will also improve cognitive function

HPA axis

A system that controls reactions to stress and regulates body processes including digestion, the immune system, mood, emotions, sexuality, and energy

Huperzine A

A nootropic that acts on the acetylcholine system and is an acetylcholinesterase inhibitor, giving it a powerful effect on cognitive function

Hypothalamus

A small portion of the brain that links the nervous system with the endocrine system

L-Theanine

An amino acid naturally found in green tea

Lemon Balm

An herb in the mint family that is native to the Mediterranean and Central Asia regions of the world. It's used for culinary flavoring and is a popular plant for distillation for use in essential oil blends.

Lion's Mane
An edible mushroom that contains a class of compounds that stimulates the production of nerve growth factor (NGF)

Magnesium
Magnesium is a cofactor, or enzyme catalyst, in more than 300 systems that regulate biochemical reactions in the body. Magnesium controls the growth of muscle tissue and regulates your energy levels. It is also required for the synthesis of DNA, RNA, and the "master antioxidant," glutathione.

Matcha
A finely ground powder made from a special kind of green tea leaves. It has many more antioxidants than standard green tea. When drinking matcha, you consume the entire leaf that is ground up and stirred into hot water, as opposed to steeping a tea bag and removing it.

Mitochondria
The powerhouse of the cell. This is where the biochemical processes of respiration and energy production occurs.

Modafinil
A wakefulness-promoting agent that is used to treat excessive sleepiness caused by sleep problems such as narcolepsy or sleep apnea

Neurotransmitters
Brain chemicals that control many of your moods, emotions, and other sensations. Scientists and researchers have identified over 100 neurotransmitters. There are two kinds of neurotransmitters, inhibitory and excitatory. You need a balance of both.

Noopept
An extremely potent nootropic that is documented to be 1,000 times stronger than piracetam. The dosage that is generally recommended in powder form is no larger than what will fit on the tip of a toothpick.

Nootropics
Drugs, supplements, nutraceuticals, and foods that can enhance your cognition and boost your brainpower

Norepinephrine

A powerful brain chemical. It acts as both a neurotransmitter and a hormone. When under significant stress, norepinephrine causes an increase in blood sugar and heart rate to ensure adequate fuel to deal with or escape a threat.

Oxiracetam

A racetam comparable to piracetam, but is more effective for memory. It has been shown to increase cognition by 1 point on a 5-point scale with no side effects whatsoever.

Panax ginseng

An herb that helps rejuvenate the body and mind. It has been found to significantly improve working memory and cognitive function.

Parasympathetic nervous system

One of two branches in the autonomic nervous system. Responsible for slowing the heart rate, increasing intestinal and glandular activity, and relaxing the sphincter muscles.

Phenylpiracetam

Similar to piracetam. A group of atoms are added to the compound piracetam to allow it to penetrate the blood-brain barrier.

Phosphatidylserine

A powerful nutrient for protecting human brain cells and enhancing overall cognitive ability

Piracetam

The "grandfather" of all nootropics. It helps boost brain function, mitochondrial function, and ATP production.

Pituitary gland

The major endocrine gland attached to the brainstem, which is important in controlling growth and development and the functioning of the other endocrine glands

Pramiracetam

A smart drug similar to piracetam and has been proven to be helpful in young males with memory and cognitive problems, specifically those suffering from head injuries in the absence of oxygen

Racetams

A family of nootropics that were discovered in 1960. Most are generally mild nootropics. They are capable of improving memory, cognitive performance, attention span, and other related markers.

Reishi

An herbal mushroom that is nontoxic and can be taken daily to regulate the immune system

Relora

A patented and proprietary blend of two separate natural compounds designed for synergy. Can help relieve anxiety.

Rhodiola rosea

Also referred to as "the golden root." It is a mood and energy-boosting compound. It's great for reducing fatigue and increasing endurance.

Serotonin

A neurotransmitter that is involved in the transmission of nerve impulses. It is also known as the "happy" chemical. It regulates mood, social behavior, appetite, and other functions such as digestion.

Serotoninergics

Supplements that work on the serotonin system

Shankpushi

An herb that can help with chronic cough, sleeplessness, epilepsy, anxiety, and more. It also possesses anti-stress, antidepressant, anti-anxiety, antioxidant, and even analgesic properties.

Stacking

Taking multiple compounds, nutrients, herbs, etc. together to enhance the effects of one another.

Sympathetic nervous system

One of the two major branches in the autonomic nervous system. It is responsible for the "fight or flight" response to stress.

Tyrosine

A synthetic nootropic category. It can be found naturally in many food sources such as fish, chicken, and pork. Tyrosine is one of many amino acids that act as a building block of protein molecules. Without enough tyrosine in the system, your thyroid can become underactive.

Vinpocetine

A health supplement that originates from the periwinkle plant

Vitamin B$_{12}$

A crucial nutrient for your nerve health and for the production of red blood cells that carry oxygen throughout your body

Vitamin D

An essential steroid hormone and immune modulator that you get primarily from either sun exposure or supplementation

Standard U.S./Metric Measurement Conversions

VOLUME CONVERSIONS

U.S. Volume Measure	Metric Equivalent
⅛ teaspoon	0.5 milliliter
¼ teaspoon	1 milliliter
½ teaspoon	2 milliliters
1 teaspoon	5 milliliters
½ tablespoon	7 milliliters
1 tablespoon (3 teaspoons)	15 milliliters
2 tablespoons (1 fluid ounce)	30 milliliters
¼ cup (4 tablespoons)	60 milliliters
⅓ cup	90 milliliters
½ cup (4 fluid ounces)	125 milliliters
⅔ cup	160 milliliters
¾ cup (6 fluid ounces)	180 milliliters
1 cup (16 tablespoons)	250 milliliters
1 pint (2 cups)	500 milliliters
1 quart (4 cups)	1 liter (about)

WEIGHT CONVERSIONS

U.S. Weight Measure	Metric Equivalent
½ ounce	15 grams
1 ounce	30 grams
2 ounces	60 grams
3 ounces	85 grams
¼ pound (4 ounces)	115 grams
½ pound (8 ounces)	225 grams
¾ pound (12 ounces)	340 grams
1 pound (16 ounces)	454 grams

OVEN TEMPERATURE CONVERSIONS

Degrees Fahrenheit	Degrees Celsius
200 degrees F	95 degrees C
250 degrees F	120 degrees C
275 degrees F	135 degrees C
300 degrees F	150 degrees C
325 degrees F	160 degrees C
350 degrees F	180 degrees C
375 degrees F	190 degrees C
400 degrees F	205 degrees C
425 degrees F	220 degrees C
450 degrees F	230 degrees C

BAKING PAN SIZES

American	Metric
8 x 1½ inch round baking pan	20 x 4 cm cake tin
9 x 1½ inch round baking pan	23 x 3.5 cm cake tin
11 x 7 x 1½ inch baking pan	28 x 18 x 4 cm baking tin
13 x 9 x 2 inch baking pan	30 x 20 x 5 cm baking tin
2 quart rectangular baking dish	30 x 20 x 3 cm baking tin
15 x 10 x 2 inch baking pan	30 x 25 x 2 cm baking tin (Swiss roll tin)
9 inch pie plate	22 x 4 or 23 x 4 cm pie plate
7 or 8 inch springform pan	18 or 20 cm springform or loose bottom cake tin
9 x 5 x 3 inch loaf pan	23 x 13 x 7 cm or 2 lb narrow loaf or pate tin
1½ quart casserole	1.5 liter casserole
2 quart casserole	2 liter casserole

Index